DEAR CANCER, LOVE STACY

Dear Cancer, Love Stacy

STACY MIDDLEMAN

POPULAR.

DEAR CANCER, LOVE STACY

ISBN   978-1-5445-0034-8   *Paperback*

978-1-5445-0035-5   *Ebook*

for Ethan and Ryan

"We are here to laugh at the odds and live life so well that death will tremble to take us."

—CHARLES BUKOWSKI

Prologue

Cancer runs in my family.

My grandfather and his seven siblings all had some form or another, disease showing up in older age. My mother's younger sister had breast cancer in her thirties. When I was twenty-seven and pregnant with my daughter, my mother was diagnosed. She was twice my age at fifty-four.

Consumed with new motherhood, I was not ready to focus on my growing risk for breast cancer, but with her diagnosis I felt a direct hit.

Three years after my daughter was born, at the age of thirty, I began getting mammograms. However premature it seemed, with my strong family history I knew I had to do something. *Be proactive.*

The summer I turned thirty-five, I had my third mammogram, and my last.

✳ ✳ ✳

The school year had just begun and I was pestered by having to go. I was a healthy young woman too busy to be bothered with unwanted appointments, but something was gnawing at me. Wishing it away, I also knew it would be foolish to ignore. Why I recall the irritation is a wonder. Not hindsight, but a nagging sensation of what was to become.

If I was shaking during the exam, it was not from nerves but the arctic temperature of the room. A nurse called me back to repeat the test and there on the film, visible to the naked eye, was a small cluster of spots on the right side of my chest. She wanted a magnification and needed to take another shot. I was shivering from the cold, too uncomfortable to sense the magnitude of her concern. And then the radiologist confirmed her distress. She said I needed to see a breast surgeon right away.

I called my husband to relay the news, more a report about my appointment than a warning. Already I was plugging my ears, making myself deaf to the siren, muting the possibility from my mind. This was a routine mammogram. I was thirty-five, a picture of health.

There was no way I could have cancer. There was no way I could have cancer yet.

* * *

My cancer was considered Stage 0 and urgency was not a driving factor. It was detected so early that a medically reasonable option was to have no treatment at all. I was told that ductal carcinoma in situ, or DCIS, can remain dormant for up to ten years and might never develop into invasive cancer.

But I wasn't taking any chances.

During those chaotic weeks of discovery, I also had genetic testing to determine if I was a carrier of the BRCA mutation, which brings with it a predisposition for developing breast and ovarian cancer, among others. The positive test result confirmed what I already knew: that my risk for disease was extremely high. By the time I received these results, my decision had already been made.

I was going to have a bilateral mastectomy, complete removal of both of my breasts.

∗   ∗   ∗

It was early fall and the Jewish holidays were approaching when I had to arrange for surgery. I scheduled the operation six weeks out, after Rosh Hashanah and Yom Kippur, to prepare myself and my family for the weeks to come.

Although my treatment wasn't pressing, our emotions were acute. The gift of time allowed us room to grieve.

I spent the better part of those weeks readying myself, exercising to keep my body strong and eating as healthfully as I could. My mother-in-law planned to stay in our home and take care of our children while I was in the hospital, then take them away to visit her family, giving us a week to recuperate without interruption. They were seven and nine at the time.

My husband would drive the kids to school in the mornings and I arranged carpools for each afternoon. I made a calendar with everyone's assignment, who would be driving my children and when: friends to drop them home from school, others to take them to and from their afternoon activities. I made playdates for weekends and informed all the teachers and staff at our school, organizing every last detail for a month in advance. Secretary of State for the state of my life.

I also started an email list to communicate with friends, family and the community that was rallying behind me. Dependent on their help, I wanted to keep them informed about my schedule as well as my progress.

Everyone who expressed their condolences and concern was added to my list. Anyone who cared.

Wading through my own confusion, I felt compelled to articulate the experience, to educate and enlighten others about what it meant to have a mastectomy. It wasn't so much about cancer—I was never in fear for my life—as it was about undergoing such a radical change, particularly at my age.

I felt a responsibility to the people around me, especially the young women in my community. The disease was more common among our tribe, Jewish women of European descent, all of us at higher risk. I had been lucky and caught it early. A cautionary tale.

I also hated gossip. If people were going to spread rumors about me, they were going to get it right. What began as a simple matter of communication grew into an expression of my experience. Turns out, I needed to share.

I've been praying to God
but it feels more like begging
This old soul of mine in a body so young

I want to live more of this
life that I'm living
To be a good mother
woman and wife

So take from my body and bury it early
then leave me alone for the
rest of my days

For my spirit is worthy
and ready to conquer

and I'll live my life fuller
in so many ways

OCTOBER 8, 2005

My surgery was successful but recovery was more difficult than we were told to expect. I was in constant pain and could not drive for seven weeks, which left me with few restful nights and plenty to talk about. I began sending emails routinely. Writing felt necessary, not because I thought I was a good writer, or a writer at all.

I just had to get things off my chest.

When the words started coming, in poetry and letters and as an outpouring of my soul, I did not know I had them until they appeared, often in the middle of the night, when many of those emails were sent. My schedule and treatment became irrelevant in relief of explaining my experience. I was sharing my life before sharing became a way of life. The release it provided, and the response from family, friends and an ever-growing list of acquaintances became my salvation.

A year and a half passed, from diagnosis to the completion of my reconstruction. My struggle began in pain but ended with what I thought was tremendous growth. I had endured. My life had been altered, my body was changed, and I had bared my soul in the process. I had lived out loud, and with it came acceptance. A new sense of self. Confidence. And wisdom.

As far as cancer was concerned, I had checked that off my list. I did what had to be done, and now I got to move on with my life.

Which is exactly what I did.

* * *

The dressing room was crowded and tiny. Discarded clothes were piling up on the floor, and it was getting hot. My daughter and I had squeezed in together, sharing the space as we shopped, when I lifted my shirt and noticed the lump. It had been there a while, a little bump below my breast, but something wasn't right. This thing had *grown*.

Eight and a half years had passed since my diagnosis.

There was no way I could have cancer.

Both of my breasts had been completely removed. I had passed the significant five-year survival mark by a long shot. I was vigilant in my care, had screenings every year, and was in great shape. I *knew* my body.

There was no way I could have cancer again.

* * *

Three weeks after my second diagnosis, after surgery to remove the lump I'd found in the dressing room, after the chaos of gathering records and meeting with doctors, after telling my family and closest friends, after a second surgery to remove the rest of the tumor, and some lymph nodes, and my ovaries, and after receiving my prognosis and treatment plan, I started a Facebook page to share with the world.

My college roommate had introduced me to Facebook. We'd been out of school for fifteen years and loosely kept in touch. By email, with birthday cards, an occasional chat on the phone. Facebook was something new, and she asked me to give it a try. I wasn't technologically savvy, but I signed up. And then I forgot about it.

By the time people started using Facebook in earnest, I had forgotten my password and couldn't access my account. Besides, people were using it for ridiculous things. Like posting their whereabouts, or what they were eating for dinner. I was not interested.

Several years passed before I updated my account and joined the masses, pressured by out-of-town friends to keep in touch the easy way. My status included the usual posts: pictures of my family, the occasional travel brag, attempts at humor and spreading information, just like everyone else. Though I'd never really begun, I was back, beginning my journey down the rabbit hole. Facebook seemed like a waste of time. Childish. For years I resisted.

And then it saved me.

Again, I felt compelled to write. And I knew I'd have to let it all out.

This is where my story begins.

Fight like a girl.

March 28, 2014

Dear Cancer,

Go fuck yourself.

Love Stacy

"You may have to fight a battle more than once to win it."

—MARGARET THATCHER

March 28, 2014

Dear Cancer,

I'm lying in bed right now, well, not anymore, just another day of not feeling good because today I spent eight hours in the hospital getting this stupid port catheter put in—my third surgery in three weeks—and it stings and hurts my neck and feels difficult to swallow, not from the inside but the outside, and yet I know, I absolutely know I will get past this. I will deal with it and get through it just like the six-hour surgery last week, the chemo happily on its way, and whatever other horrors still beckon, because none of this compares to what has been the most painful of all of these ridiculous experiences. What hurts more than any-thing, more than the double mastectomy which kept me on prescription pain meds for sixty-six straight days back in 2005, or the reconstruction whereby saline injections were used to stretch out my chest for months, or the five IVs—no, six, because the nurse had to take one out and start over—I've had in the last month, or the countless blood tests and PET scans and X-rays, or the face-down MRI which caused my upwardly positioned arms to go numb, worse than the dread of gadolinium dye or radioactive sugar or nuclear medicine injected somewhere in the one millimeter of tissue between my skin and implant, or the major excision to my right side or the lymph node dissection under my arm (that fucking hurts) or the four holes punched into my abdomen to pluck out my healthy little ovaries that were stealthily feeding my cancer, more than any of this was the realization, the very, very real understanding that my life could possibly end. I don't mean that loosely existential fear we all have of dying. Not that subconscious, ignorant, far off feeling that most of us are really never willing to acknowledge anyway: that no one gets out alive. I'm talking about Way Too Soon. Before My Time. I'm talking about a life, a beautiful, happy, full of love life stolen: missing graduations and weddings and grandbabies and anniversaries, and even more than all that, the idea of not being there for my children when they one day face their demons, life crises that sadly may mirror my own.

I have received enough information to be able to escape that black hole of fear. I had only let it in a little at a time and just once was utterly overcome. And it will never entirely go away. That is the difference between the first time and now. But I am ready for the fight. And some sleep.

Love Stacy

"What fresh hell is this?"

—DOROTHY PARKER

March 28, 2014

Dear Cancer,

An amazing thing happened: the throbbing soreness under my arm that's been debilitating me for days just suddenly disappeared, chased away by the shrieking pain in my chest from the port. Every victory counts!

Love Stacy

Cancer

June 22 — July 22

Think twice before debating with
a Cancer, their passion makes
them very fearsome opponents.

March 28, 2014

Dear Cancer,

I'm a Cancer, too.

Love Stacy

"If you have good thoughts they will shine out of your face like sunbeams and you will always look lovely."
—ROALD DAHL

March 28, 2014

Dear Cancer,

These hot flashes I'm getting, night sweats really, have absolutely nothing to do with you. I'm just HOT. Period.

Love Stacy

"We're all just walking each other home."
—RAM DASS

March 30, 2014

Dear Cancer,

Tonight Dave and I went out for the first (and possibly last) time in a long while. It was a beautiful night and I felt great—I had to sport the new do before it's shortly gone— and we ran into several friends whom we love, at some of the places we have loved during our life here. Which got me thinking about how there are so many people who may not be a part of my daily life but are still such a special part of my life, which is one of the reasons I felt compelled to reach out like I do: not with some narcissistic desire for attention but to share that part of me that has received your love, or understanding, or admiration (and vice versa), from so many of you over the years. People who have had an impact on me, whether it was eight years ago, or eighteen, or twenty-eight. And it made me realize there are two things, and maybe—probably—only two things, that heal: time and love. The very conditions that are most precious

and consequently cannot be touched, or bought, or clearly
defined for that matter. Which makes me feel, in some
small way, that I've got it all figured out.

Love Stacy

Cut and removed
Sliced and observed
Noted, discarded, the end

Those were my breasts
From my God-given body
That is material, my friend

Not jewelry or shoes
Clothing nor cars
Homes and their furnishings, too

Why do we care for innocuous things
When we're given our body in health

The love that we give to
our family and friends
And the joy we receive in return

That is material by which
we should measure
Our lives and the meaning of wealth

NOVEMBER 3, 2005

When life hands you lemons
make grape juice.

Then sit back and watch as the
world wonders how you did it.

March 31, 2014

Dear Cancer,

Watch me.

Love Stacy

I love you so much, I will even talk to you on the phone.[1]

March 31, 2014

Dear Cancer,

I know I started all this by first asking people not to call. It is true, in the beginning of a crisis like this, there is literally no time to spare for anything less than what is the urgent task at hand. Contacting family, calling medical offices, consulting with doctors, transferring records, coordinating appointments, juggling life in such a way that busy people—those who make "busy" an occupation—would never understand. It's an unjust metaphor, but somehow, happily, reminds me of the time I came home from the hospital with my first-born Ethan, and was so exhausted and consumed with nursing and changing diapers, and breathing, that I had no time to eat or shower, or the other way around, so David made me a sandwich and brought it to me while I was taking a bath. It was the best peanut

---

1   Text sourced from illustration by someecards.com

butter and jelly I have ever had, mostly because I remember it seventeen and a half years later. I digress.

Understand, I had to protect my phone lines the way one would guard the Hope Diamond. And we never had caller ID until the first time we went through this, when we were equally overwhelmed by the outpouring of support as we were totally consumed with making arrangements. As the last holdouts, we were forced to distinguish friendly calls from incoming doctors and hospitals.

Do not misunderstand: if anyone wants to reach me, who knows me enough to want to call, by all means, do. I decided decades ago that I control the phone and not the other way around. If I am not available, I don't answer. If I don't want to be available, I don't answer. In fact, that is how I learned to weed out less-than-genuine friends, the ones who, when cell phones came into fashion, were puzzlingly unavailable to me but would never miss a beat with the crowd, of which I have never, nor will ever want to be a part. And still, I believe in the prerogative of selectivity, not as a method of manipulation but as a tool to keep my life in balance. It's called taking control. And it's okay.

And if you're hoping to just leave a message, we never answer during dinner.

I start chemo on Thursday and probably need a week to adjust, so please be respectful. But call all you want, if you want. If you love me, you know who you are. And if you don't know who you are, take my word for it, it's time to figure that out.

Love Stacy

laughing, though I do it, hurts
crying, though I may,
hurts worse
sneezing is so painful that
although I must, I hold at bay

these little joys and itches, too
so natural and so needed
I can't control although I've tried
imagine how I've pleaded

so do not take the little things
you have in life
for granted
for one day you may wake up, too
and find your life has slanted

NOVEMBER 24, 2005

"Things turn out best for those who make the best of the way things turn out."
—JACK BUCK

March 31, 2014

Dear Cancer,

Thank you all, every one of you, for your incredible response to me, my journey, my words ... I cannot possibly acknowledge the thousands of likes, comments, messages sent my way, but please know I am receiving—and appreciating— every single one.

I am a bit overwhelmed right now with my pre-medication schedule, and will be out of commission for a few days working on a tangible and very exciting project at the heart of my long and happy future, but I'll be back.

I will be back.

Love Stacy

"Life isn't about waiting for the storm to pass. It's about learning to dance in the rain."

—VIVIAN GREENE

April 2, 2014

Dear Cancer,

I am getting ready for chemo tomorrow, plainly not a minute to spare, and yet I feel compelled to write. Not to document my every move—surely this will be there for the recollection—but because part of my consumption are the thoughts constantly spinning through my mind. I have so much going on right now, not just getting through the treatment, but living my life. Spending time, passing moments really, with my family, attempting to have meals together as we always do, but feeling scattered by the ever constant of what's next. Evenings magically disappear, and my kids and I seem to be ships passing in the night, though fairly attributed to the fact that they are teenagers, who seem to be doing just fine, occupying themselves in their usual studious and social ways. The other night when we had the pep talk about this upcoming week, and I promised things should resume to normal hopefully soon, my son Ethan said everything feels normal now. My daughter Ryan, on the other hand—a newly appointed driver—just wants her own car. Apparently I have not only braced myself, but these miraculously strong and impervious children as well. I wonder often how this will affect them, not just now but in the long run: in the scheme of their own lives and how they will learn to cope. I expect well, and I expect to be there to support them.

I have not been inside a grocery store nor prepared a single dinner in the past month—I have the world's best house husband, seriously—though I've kept up with endless laundry and general chores, banal luxuries in a life kept simple, finding joy in the small things and appreciation for everything. I have help for the heavy stuff, but I don't mind taking care of my home. It is my sacred space. Beds will be made, dirty clothes will be cleaned and put away, my house will be in order because it has to be, stupid cancer or otherwise. My mother used to shrewdly say, "cleanliness is close to godliness." Our styles may differ, but it was one of those things that stuck, and is exactly what I will come home to find tomorrow: a place of peace. It is both an effortless and exalted way in which we choose to live.

So this evening, while I scurry about my house, with no time for even a last-minute call to my parents or dearest of friends, it is because I am setting a thermometer at bedside to regularly check for fever, beware the greatest risk, infection; making charts for the complicated schedule of medicines administered at home, a five-day regimen surrounding chemo. I am packing reading and writing materials, music and electronics, flotsam and jetsam to pass the time because I have no idea how I will feel during the six hours of being tethered to an IV. I've been advised to bring a blanket or scarf to cover the bags in case I don't care to see the toxic poisons, in all manner of dazzling colors, dripping ever so slowly into tiny little me. Gathering snacks and drinks, and crushed and bagged ice to chew on so I don't get sores in my mouth. And not an effort made on David's behalf. He is on his own and in accord. I'm really not scared, shocking as the many side effects may be. They are to be anticipated but not expected, which is exactly my approach. And though our experiences may vary, my father has always imparted that "this too shall pass." Wise words instilled, indeed.

Love Stacy

Be the kind of woman that when your feet hit the floor each morning, the devil says, "Oh crap, she's up!" [2]

April 3, 2014

Dear Cancer,

Here we go. Let's get her done.

Science, you do your job. Spirit, I'll do mine.

Love Stacy

---

2 Uncredited; adapted from the quote by Joanne Clancy: "Be the kind of woman who, when your feet hit the floor each morning, the devil says, 'Oh no, she's up!'"

"Don't save something for a special occasion. Every day of your life is a special occasion."

—THOMAS S. MONSON

April 3, 2014

Dear Cancer,

Today was not so bad at all, and then Dave bestowed upon me the most beautiful gift, an heirloom to stand the test of time—incidentally purchased before my diagnosis, coincidentally arriving now—that will forever commemorate not this day but every day of life we share together.

Little chemo, big therapy, and eternal love.

Love Stacy

"Nothing ever goes away until it teaches us what we need to know."

—PEMA CHODRON

April 4, 2014

Dear Cancer,

I would never accuse myself of being stubborn. Persistent, determined, uncompromising? You bet. Obstinate, unyielding, inflexible? Absolutely not. I am highly adaptable, adjusting easily to any circumstance and dealing with it accordingly. Case in point. Part of being flexible is recognizing your flaws, accepting your mistakes—and not beating yourself up about it. But if there is one thing I have learned from this second diagnosis, it has been my profound arrogance. Wholly blindsided, never did I believe this would happen. Ever. Again.

My doctors were equally puzzled, shocked to be fair, and when we first met with my oncologist she was patently frustrated, continually referring to my case as being "outside the box." Normally I would take that as a compliment, but now? Not so much. She presented my situation to Tumor Board, a gathering by which thirty doctors or so, of varying areas of expertise, meet to discuss unusual cases. It is meant to be a learning opportunity but also a method by which to form a consensus on how to proceed with a confounding set of circumstances. Combined with our numerous family and friends in the medical field, no less than four dozen doctors and one very special pharmacist have been privy to this event. Barring my condition, that made me feel pretty fucking special. But back to my arrogance ...

Not long ago I read an article online about the habits of people with common sense. Pouring down the list, patting myself on the back as I confidently checked off each attribute as my own—things like setting boundaries, not poisoning your body or spending money you don't have, building friendships for genuine, meaningful connection rather than to benefit yourself, and not making excuses for people—a note or two struck a deeper chord. Having goals and planning for the future while still being flexible because unexpected setbacks may arise? Sure, proof positive. But here's the kicker: knowing it's okay to change one's mind...

Stubbornness and close-mindedness aren't virtues. People with good sense are able to objectively assess situations and see different viewpoints, giving themselves the freedom to change their opinions when they have more information. That's called learning and having humility.[3]

Well, hell if I haven't learned something and embraced humility. All these years of vigilance, to say nothing of acknowledging my family history by starting mammograms at thirty and discovering cancer at thirty-five, enduring the double mastectomy which served to both eradicate on one side and prevent on the other, reducing my chances of recurrence significantly, like, maybe, forever. What's a girl to do?

Here's what: wake up and remember there are no guarantees in life, ever. Accept that life isn't fair but worth the taking, and take absolutely nothing for granted.

Love Stacy

---

3   Victoria Fedden, "The 12 Habits of People with Good Sense," Elephant Journal, January 6, 2014, accessed April 4, 2014, https://www.elephantjournal. com/2014/01/the-top-12-habits-of-people-with-good-sense/

For those of you who wish your breasts
were larger or uplifted

For those of you who wish that
body weight could just be shifted

For those of you who wish for
lesser wrinkles on your brow

For those of you who count the years
and think to yourself — how?

If you are one who deprecates
yourself and all you have
Always wanting something changed
or always wanting more

Stop for just a moment please
And think about your body
If it's not diseased and doesn't hurt
You have nothing else to wish for

JANUARY 5, 2006

After Tuesday, even the calendar goes WTF

April 5, 2014

Dear Cancer,

Uh-oh, here it comes. The bone pain from yesterday's Neulasta shot to keep up my white count, forcing my bone marrow to work overtime and therefore rendering me a worthless pile of, I don't know, not me. The first night was less than terrible, just a generalized feeling of yuck, not quite nausea, but an awareness to not let that feeling go too far—I have an arsenal of prescriptions to ward it off even though the first IV bag in a series of plenty was a drug to do just that, but with the proficiency of lasting five full days in my system. So I was thrilled when I did not have to resort to the expected regimen of Zofran and Phenergen that would undeniably wreak havoc on my poor tummy that is already a wading pool of tablets and toxins.

Yesterday came on the generalized bitchiness, but that had nothing to do with chemo at all. Some hack in San

Antonio tried to tap into my Gmail account forcing me to change my password, which is something I am actually capable of technologically figuring out on my own, but one thing led to another, and the computer stopped sharing my calendar with my phone, and well, that is when all hell broke loose. It took me the better part of the whole damn day to get that one taken care of and—*Surprise!*—I have better things to do with my time. Like take an occasional unpleasant shower and change my bandages, still necessary until Sunday when ten days have passed from the port catheter incisions, lest we forget the acute and fundamental responsibility of sitting around waiting for this chemo business to rear its ugly head.

Last night I even had a hot flash. A real, live, I-cannot-cool-off moment that had nothing to do with being buried under my covers like a hibernating bear, which is actually how I sleep almost every night of the year, and especially so in warm climates, when David, who can't stand the weight of the down comforter he purchased so very long ago, folds it over to my side, so I get double the pleasure and triple the night sweats I've had for the past decade, which come to think of it, may have had nothing to do with being peri-menopausal in the first place, as I was classified several years back, though I am now in fact really-menopausal, as instantly granted from surgery to remove my ovaries three weeks ago.

I'm not precisely sure what is happening right now. I think mostly I just can't sleep—lots of unfavorable effects from the armory of drugs used to deflect the more adversarial ones. And since it's only midnight, tomorrow is a whole new day.

Love Stacy

Nope.[4]

April 7, 2014

Warning: You have been warned.

Dear Cancer,

I would be remiss ... No.

I would be a total fraud if I didn't acknowledge that something in me broke this weekend. I have never known suffering like this before. And I have known suffering. I have never felt like I couldn't do this, until this weekend when I felt like I cannot do this again. I have never felt like this isn't worth it, until I realized that to live like this ... is ... not ... worth it. For the first time in my life, I recognized, admitted, I don't know what, that if this ever happens again—if this cancer comes back ... in two years, in ten—I will not fight it. I will not live to suffer. I will not survive just to die. Quality of life is so much more important than quantity. It's not a race. Who cares who lives the longest? I want to live fully. Happily. Meaningfully. I do not want to be miserable. That is not an acceptable existence. I do not

---

4   Text sourced from illustration by Gemma Correll.

want my family to be miserable. *That* is not an acceptable existence. Having someone around who is suffering, and only suffering, does not make life better for anyone. That is NOT A LIFE. And it's not going to be mine.

I cannot even begin to describe what it was that I just went through. There are no words to articulate how incomprehensible it was, and I'm pretty tough. And not weak with words. I am okay enough to write about it now, but it has taken all of me to get here. I was absolutely, totally, and completely incapacitated this weekend. I could not move. I couldn't turn my head without severe vertigo, tipping over like a weeble-wobble. I could barely make it to the bathroom, and only did so when forced, and only if accompanied. When I spoke to the on-call doctor, she asked if it felt like I was spinning or if the room was spinning, and I could not make the distinction. I experienced not acute pain, but an ache so deep, it was on a cellular level: every single cell, from the top of my head to the tips of my toes, hurt in such a way that I could feel every single one. Time remained at a standstill. Every moment was extensive. The night felt like days and the days felt like a week. Not from boredom, anguish perhaps; but a truly metaphysical distortion. I would check the clock, and if thirty minutes had passed, I had thought it two hours. For twenty-four hours I lay in bed wondering how on earth I will be able to do this again, and again. And again. And then thinking, after that, never again.

Since this all began, in August of 2005, I have had five surgeries and nineteen incisions. Yes: I have been cut NINE-TEEN times. And I'm not done. Oh, and I neglected the needle biopsy where it all began, which seems so benign—buried so deeply below the enormous pile of shit I've been through that I almost forgot. It wasn't benign. At all. It was fucking cancer. And it hurt. Another one of those face-down exams where a needle was directed, precisely by computer, to be shot like a gun—an actual sniper into my breast—to target the very specific site of suspicion. And then the recoveries, and the drains, and the exams, and the scans. It is endless. Positively fucking interminable.

It's been five weeks so far. That's it. I have twelve weeks to go. Then possibly radiation. If radiation, then probably reconstruction. And I've been down that road ... I mean more reconstruction. I can no longer remember the last time I drove my car. Or checked the mail. Or saw my kids off to school in the morning. I haven't walked my dogs but once. And they're dachshunds. They know. I can't remember when I last felt any physical pleasure, and I'm not getting personal. Well, actually, this is very personal. But I'm talking about the basics. I hug my kids because I love them, but it doesn't feel good. I shower because I have to. But it is not pleasant. The skin on my chest is shredded from adhesives I had to use to keep the port covered for ten days, and the port ... oh my god, it is absolutely horrible. It's like having two nickels stacked together and shoved under my skin. On my chest. Already pulled so tight and thin. And the taste in my mouth? That's the least of it. Just don't brush your teeth for a month and you'll see. No, I'll go easy: try it for a week. And you can floss, because, *ew*, you can't not floss. It's not metallic, so much. Just gross.

And next I lose my hair.

I have not wanted to do anything. Not a thing. I didn't want to talk to anyone. I couldn't look at the computer, or turn on the TV, or even hold a book. I wondered if this is what it's like to be depressed. 'Cause I've been down, but not like this. I hate depressives. Depression is boring. And so I questioned whether I would end up being forever more compassionate, or never feeling compassion again.

Anyway, I'm going to be okay, and this is depressing. But I feel better now. You may not, but I do. So here, I'll turn it around for you.

Go outside. Take a walk. Maybe you'll see a puppy. Or a rainbow.

Love Stacy

"Write what should not be forgotten."

—ISABEL ALLENDE

April 8, 2014

Dear Cancer,

Yeah, I know. That last one was really heavy. But I am so much better today.

Love Stacy

Your life is your message to the world.
Make sure it's inspiring.

April 11, 2014

Dear Cancer,

I have been meaning to write, overwhelmed of late with emotion and opportunity, profound perspective, both the goodness and bad of all this; friends old and new sharing stories of pain and suffering, triumph and love, and I am so, so grateful. I began this as a selfish catharsis; that is all. But if I am reaching anyone, that turns around and reaches me back. So thank you.

I have so much going on right now, both physically and on my mind. Our life's pendulum swings violently, from David's retirement—his great and well-deserved success— to my shocking and unexpected diagnosis, one having absolutely nothing to do with the other, yet culminating at precisely the same time. His departure, pending for six months, finally closed on the day of and during my six-hour surgery.

We are so blessed, and in love, and so full of love and good fortune. Yet there is balance, a striking and delicate one at that. I had several "good" days this week, good being less illustrative than somewhat normal. I was able to get out, practice yoga, be about half-way productive until the early afternoons when I needed to rest, and then on Thursday experienced another setback, almost a relapse if you will. I was again debilitated by aching joints, a constant headache, and now spasms in my spine. Something is doing me in.

But I have so much to look forward to, accomplishments to be made, and everyday life to be lived. A future so exciting and broad, it is often difficult to contain, and dare I say confounded by fear that this disease is hunting me down. Worry not, I refuse to let that get the better of me. I just need to speak my truth.

Love Stacy

"The brave may not live forever but the cautious do not live at all."

—MEG CABOT

April 13, 2014

Dear Cancer,

Well, I'll be damned but today I feel like a million bucks. One hundred percent. If I continue to feel like this until my next treatment, I'll be just fine. I am going to be fabulous anyway, but maybe, hopefully, not so bothered by the next three rounds. Eleven days down.

And if timing is everything, my next task is to shave my head. The chemo is generous enough to provide a warning. My scalp will begin to tingle and become tender, but when the hair starts falling, it comes out en masse, and I'm not going to that party. I don't know exactly when, but when is soon, and I have people to see and places to go, so I'll be fitting in this thing-to-do shortly.

A few weeks ago I tried on wigs—test that for an afternoon of entertainment—but no luck. My head is so small (which, I guess, is better than the alternative) that most were way too cumbersome for my face. If I decide later that I want one, it will have to be custom made. I think I'll be content with all the hats and scarves I've collected, but once again, a new experience, and I have no idea how that light will shine until I've walked through the tunnel.

I give my family twenty-four hours to adjust before they start cracking the jokes. And I'm fine with that. I am going to be great fodder.

Love Stacy

Life is better when you're laughing.

April 15, 2014

Dear Cancer,

Today we were supposed to depart for London, our first spring break together in three years. Just the four of us, for eight days. I have never been. There is nothing I love more than to be alone, away, with my family. Unplugged, disconnected, and therefore totally reconnected. It is my favorite thing to do: to see the world, but even more enjoyably, to watch as my children see the world. I have always lived with the mantra: *minds wide open*. That is how I raise my kids. I want them to explore the world, beyond their school, their neighborhood, this city or state or country. I want them to experience other cultures and architecture and food, and to understand that nearly no one lives with the kind of privilege they have known.

But back to why I love our travels so much is the memories we have created along the way. Some of our funniest family moments have occurred on trips, and it never seems to matter where we are. In Costa Rica several years ago, the kids were picking up coconuts on the beach. They must have spent hours breaking into one—in their natural state, those nuts are layered and tough—and then feeling compelled to taste the fruit after such an accomplishment. Ryan was chewing on the meat, clearly not enjoying it, and as she was letting it just fall out of her mouth, she proclaimed to David, "It tastes like coconut." Don't ask why, but he laughed until he cried. He could barely breathe, it was so deadpan funny. And contagious. And Ethan, climbing up the rocky side of a waterfall at the end of a long hike, attempted to jump out into the fall but instead slipped, and went sliding and bumping his way down into the reservoir below. Looking like a cartoon, he fell without getting hurt and kept us laughing for the entire afternoon.

This past winter we were in Portugal, then Spain, on a long walk home from La Sagrada Familia in Barcelona, the phenomenal Gaudi church still under construction after more than a hundred years. Dave and I were walking hand in hand, the kids in step behind us. I turned to look, and Ethan had taken Ryan's hand; they were clearly suppressing giggles while mimicking us. I then put my arm around David, and Ethan followed suit. So I put my hand in David's back pocket, and that is when Ethan exclaimed, mockingly, "Mom, you're making this uncomfortable for me." Nevertheless, they reached into each other's pockets, and we were all cracking up. It was a moment I will never forget, not only because it was truly hilarious but an acknowledgment that my kids get it. They are growing up in a loving home, and for that I am so grateful. It is our greatest gift, and what I live for.

It was on this trip when I noticed an enlarged mass under my right breast, but I will still remember it for our wonderful time together.

I could number the cities and name all the countries we have traveled to as a family, but the memories are countless. So London will wait. We will try again, and it will be all the sweeter for having this behind us.

Love Stacy

"How bold one gets when one is sure of being loved."

—SIGMUND FREUD

April 16, 2014

Dear Cancer,

Dave shaved his head, beat me to it. The gift of solidarity and laughter, and *Oh shit, that's what I'm going to look like!* And then, last night, what do you know? The Brazilian came first. Thanks, chemo!! Best side effect ever.

Love Stacy

Have no fear.

April 16, 2014

Dear Cancer,

All that fretting over hats and scarves and … actually, I look pretty darn cute. Bald, bold and beautiful, baby! My very close friend, who happens to be my hairstylist, has been on call the last several days, and I was surrounded by a few of my besties, plus Dave stopped by when it was all done. It was surprisingly no big deal. Maybe chemo is my kryptonite. There were no tears, which makes me sort of superhuman. Or maybe I'm just over it. But I think it's simply me living my life, knowing this is just one of the rides in my particular amusement park. It was actually kind of fun.

And I'm gonna work it.

Love Stacy

"People will stare. Make it worth their while."

—HARRY WINSTON

April 20, 2014

Dear Cancer,

Dave and I were out this weekend, in restaurants and bars, with fantastic friends, each time arriving au natural: no scarves, no hats, no inhibition. We could have passed as cult members or too-old-to-be hipsters, but instead we were just badass. I still have a tiny buzz though I suspect it will soon be true alopecia—a siren warned so I heeded it. And while I admit that it was easier to head out with Dave bald and by my side, it still took some nerve. Part of me felt beautiful, and fairly so, but the rest of me feels rightly like I just don't give a fuck. Which is pretty much what happens when you are dealing with this sort of thing, particularly the second and more serious time around. Everything that isn't really important just slips away. This is about my LIFE, my SURVIVAL, and having hair or how I look just doesn't even register on the scale of what matters anymore. Stripped down to the bare essentials, but hey, I wear it well.

Love Stacy

First learn the rules. Then break them.

April 22, 2014

Dear Cancer,

Fuck chemo. I just went to hot yoga and it felt GREAT!

Love Stacy

*"You never know how strong you are
until being strong is your only choice."*

—BOB MARLEY

April 23, 2014

Dear Cancer,

Here we go again: the drug regimen associated with chemo.
Steroids, laxatives, antihistamine, anti-inflammatory, anti-
nausea, and anti-anxiety (optional). Yes, I have a choice!
One choice: to fight this fucking disease. Me combating
the chemo that's battling the cancer that's attacking me.
It's all out warfare. And I am going to win.

Love Stacy

"Every time you find some humor in a difficult situation, you win."

—SUE FITZMAURICE

April 23, 2014

Dear Cancer,

I am shedding now. Like a little puppy dog. My hair is so short that it's not a problem, and it's not coming out all at once. Just when my head grazes against something, like a scarf, or a towel, or my hand. Dave's been making fun of me not for having *no* hair, but for not having lost it yet. I made a preemptive strike last week; I wasn't taking any chances. That's not to say I don't take risks. I just like to think I choose them responsibly. Isn't that what life is all about?

I can't tell if my head is tingling, as it is supposed to do; maybe the slight irritation is from my rubbing it too much. It feels funny, and I'm trying to figure out what's going on, which I think is normal when going through any sort of change. Awareness. Experience. Acceptance. Maybe even some Joy. Because change, most certainly, is what life is all about.

Love Stacy

"Beauty is simply reality seen with the eyes of love."

—RABINDRANATH TAGORE

April 24, 2014

Dear Cancer,

I should be sleeping right now but the pre-med steroid is jacking me up and stealing my slumber. Thus I picked up a book I set on my nightstand a few weeks ago to intentionally read—again—during this trial. *Tiny Beautiful Things* by Cheryl Strayed. I read the first chapter, and then this ...

I'm telling you, if you have any interest in staring humanity in the face—if you have any humanity at all—I encourage you to read this book. Not because it has anything to do with cancer, or with my cancer, although somehow it does. For the reason that eight and a half years ago I started writing, because I was thirty-five years old, and fuck, I had cancer, and I needed to write. I was propelled to do something, to get it off my chest if you will, to connect with family and friends ... and myself. A visceral force to live out loud.

It was authentic and candid and sometimes raw, but it was also lovely and poetic and written the way I wanted it to be read. Not disingenuous, nor insincere, just written like I wrote, the way I thought and felt at the time, but not necessarily the way I speak or behave or exist. And this time it is. More raw, equally real, often profane, and it's all the fucking truth. It is who I am, love it or leave it.

So when I read this book *Tiny Beautiful Things* last year, or maybe in 2012 when it was published, not only was I moved, over and over and over again, or saw in those pages everyone I know and love, or don't, including myself, I kept thinking: I love this girl, this woman, this writer, this human. She *writes* like I *think*! She is raw and real and compassionate, full of love and honesty and wisdom. She gets life down to its bitter and exhilarating core. She digs deep and exhumes no bullshit. Which is exactly the kind of person I want to know, to respect, to admire, to love, and to be.

Seize this treasure. Read it, relate to it, love and laugh and cry and FEEL. I never give myself the gift of re-reading a book; there are always so many more that await. But I am going to savor this one, take it all in a second time, maybe as a small nod to the metaphor of having cancer, twice.

I originally ordered it along with her then-newly released and now best-selling book, soon-to-be movie *Wild* (another beautiful examination if you set your eyes to any manuscript at all) and accidentally or otherwise was lucky enough to read *Tiny Beautiful Things* first, so by the time I read *Wild* I felt like I already knew her. And, Cheryl Strayed, one day I hope I will.

Love Stacy

I just want to spend the rest of my life laughing.

April 24, 2014

Dear Cancer,

Although my children are privy to these posts, I rarely use profanity around them, and never spoke carelessly when they were young. I take my responsibility as a parent very seriously, even more so now, as they are becoming adults. But we are evolving as a family, and as they grow and we begin to understand each other, we must continue to guide but can no longer control them.

So when Ryan uses abbreviations for everything, especially inappropriate language, it is pretty freaking funny. She keeps it wholesome with her very own urban dictionary of acronyms, such as the short form: af—*as fuck*. Dave's best friend, childless but close with my kids, was visiting one day, trying to decipher their teen lingo. His guess? Ass fucker.

An interpretation, for example: Annoying *as fuck*. Or ...

Annoying *ass fucker*. Where, my dear, grown, adult male friend has your mind been? Wait, that's superfluous. Forget "grown."

We maintain our efforts, with all our might, to exhibit positive role modeling. But not … no, never—at the expense of some good clean fun.

Love Stacy

Put up a fucking fight for what you love.

April 24, 2014

Dear Cancer,

Before I learned whether this very aggressive, high-grade, considerably large tumor had or had not invaded the rest of my body—lymph nodes, maybe; spine, a scan scare; ovary, doubtful but another red flag—amidst all the ignoring and praying and hoping, and forcing myself to believe, to be brave and fearless and chock full of courage, I was confronted with the very real and mind-blowing possibility that I would be leaving behind my family. My husband, who is the strongest man I know but would be rubble without me, and my not-quite-adult and definitely-not-yet-fully-formed children. To say nothing of our parents, having to bury not one, but for my beloved in-laws, two of their children, and siblings, extended family and friends who would surely mourn as well.

When we learn of someone's great loss or devastating illness, one thing is universal: we can't help but try to measure the tragedy. Is it worse for a parent to lose a newborn or young child whom they knew for only a short time, or for a young child to lose a mother or father or sibling whom, maybe, they will only remember from pictures or stories but never really know, hopefully living a full and happy and somehow new life? Or for a parent to lose a teenager or young adult child, whom they knew so well and loved so deeply, never getting to see them grow to their full potential, confounded by the loss of future grandchildren and further generations?

Or for a teenager or young man or woman on the cusp of becoming an adult to lose their parent, and not one, but sometimes both? I have known, intimately, every one of these survivors, dearly loved friends and family, David and myself included; souls who have suffered and endured, and whom will never ever forget. There is no appraisal for loss. It is experienced differently by everyone, but profound grief if encountered is borne, in some immeasurable way, forever.

I know I will survive this. I have faith and good medical reason to believe in my doctor's "curative intent." No promises, but strong, solid, and possibly quantifiable hope. I have rationalized what it would mean for me to perish, in the next two or ten or twenty years. Even joked about it. But any of it is too soon, and not acceptable. I am not ready. Dave is not ready. My children, who don't know it yet, will never be ready.

I love them so desperately that I would do anything to prevent their suffering. And yet they will suffer. Just not on account of me.

Love Stacy

"Nothing is permanent in this wicked world, not even our troubles."

—CHARLIE CHAPLIN

April 25, 2014

Dear Cancer,

Oh man, I feel like crap. And boy would I welcome one of those. All these drugs in my system, and there are no less than ten at the moment, completely shut me down, just as they did the first time. My personal grapes of wrath. I have three more prescriptions from which to choose, my nightstand littered with pill bottles in the most mocking presentation of clutter. And those mysterious hot flashes, striking and fleeting and real. Then tomorrow the dreaded Neulasta shot.

I am dizzy and disoriented, stumbling to my computer. Even capturing this has been a struggle. I'm making so many mistakes, easily correctible on a keyboard, but frustratingly laughable. It's like typing class in eighth grade where I cried during drills. Yep, some of you dear old friends may remember that. And please, have a laugh at my expense, for my how I've grown. I have fucking cancer for the second time, and I've barely shed a tear. But in middle school, I just couldn't get it right. How very far I have come.

I've been lying in bed with one eye open to elude the waves of nausea, a feeling I was somehow fortunate enough to avoid the last go-round, and trying to inhale deeply through it, though my breathing is labored, too. All normal side effects, if you dare call any of this normal. It is not. It's total fucking insanity. But by the grace of getting through, of moving forward, if ever so slowly, it is temporary.

Sleep evades me. Two more doses of the steroid and then I will hopefully pass out in a fit of exhaustion. When this all began, I asked if they could just put me under for six months and wake me when it's over. Request denied. So I will keep on trucking, maybe do some fucking, for "vagina rest" is over tomorrow, now six weeks post-surgery. I am bald and bitchy, *dazed and confused*, and "I'd like to quit thinking of the present, like right now, as some minor, insignificant preamble to somethin' else." What I need "... is some good ol' worthwhile visceral experience."[5]

And I'm getting it.

Love Stacy

---

5   *Dazed and Confused*, directed by Richard Linklater (Gramercy Pictures, 1993).

*"The only person you are destined to
become is the person you decide to be."*

—RALPH WALDO EMERSON

April 26, 2014

Dear Cancer,

I've been digging into the old stuff, reading the poem I
wrote on October 8, 2005, ten days before my bilateral
mastectomy. The ordeal began in late August, my diagnosis official just after Labor Day, but the risk to my health
was not imminent so I gave myself six weeks to prepare
for surgery; to process and mourn my loss, to ready my
children, to brace myself for permanent and life-altering
change. I was barely thirty-five.

And on that day those words pulled me out of bed early in
the morning, with an urgency to beg for mercy. To whom-
ever or whatever it was I reached, those pleas were not
answered. You are back, invading my body, my mind, my life.

But oh no, not my spirit. That, *that* is forever mine. *I* answered those prayers. *I* built myself back up. *I* honored my own strength and courage and character. It was my determination and fortitude and ESSENCE that brought me to this place, to be a good mother, woman and wife. To live my life to its fullest.

And nothing is stopping me now.

Love Stacy

Welcome to the shit show.

April 26, 2014

Dear Cancer,

Oh my god, I feel like total fucking shit right now. I'm trying not to say "oh my god" or "fuck" so much, but it's about the only teeny tiny thing that feels sort of semi-shitty good. It's not from nausea or diarrhea or constipation. Or even pain. It's just total fucking shit.

Which makes me feel bad or sad or something because if someone were to ask me, in two months or two years, or two thousand years from now how they will get through chemo, I will have to lie and tell the truth and say you will get through it, just like everyone before me said I would get through it, but it's going to really fucking suck. I couldn't even comprehend what that meant, and I will not be able to articulate it to the next sorry soul, other than to say that it's going to really fucking suck. You will feel like total fucking shit. But you will get through it.

Because I am, and I will, and I only have to do it two more

times, and in a few days I will be able to say I will only have to do it once more, if I choose to look at the big picture and realize I am halfway through. It's still two more times, but it's also halfway through.

Total fucking shit. Shit, shit, shit, shit, shit.

Love Stacy

If I could leave my body
for just a single day
I could leave behind this burden
all the misery of today

If I could leave my body
for just a single night
I could sleep in peace and comfort
bedding down without such fright

If I could leave my body
for just a single hour
I could clean myself without the view
of entering the shower

If I could leave my body for
just a single minute
I could feel no pain or agony
envisioning the finish

If I could leave my body
and have my old one back
I would not be who I've become
perspective I would lack

But it's peaceful to envision
the freedom I would gain
If I could leave my body
as if it were unchanged

JANUARY 17, 2006

I have nothing to complain about.

April 27, 2014

Dear Cancer,

I want for nothing. I mean, I could use some sleep, and I look forward to having my good health back. And some hair, though I'm kind of channeling Lupita Nyong'o these days because every time I see a black woman with a closely cropped cut, I think they are stunning, even though I'm as white as a summer cloud. I've bought myself two Alexander McQueen scarves because I think they are gorgeous and funny and apropos with the skulls all over them and I've been eyeing a hot pink one; and there's a painting I love but recently bought one by the same artist for David and he's just not that into another, and if it really belongs in my home it will find its way here one day like so many other great pieces before it.

But besides all that, I have everything I need. For some strange, odd, mysterious reason, I have joy. I feel happy. I am loved. My children (and their friends) have been amazing to me, so supportive and loving and unfrightened or fazed.

I have a husband who is crazy for me, even in my pitiful state, and even though I actually do complain. Sometimes.

When we moved into this house, nearly twelve years ago, it seemed large. It is, though we have grown into it beautifully. Still then, I always sensed this odd cartoonish vision of the windows bellowing out, so full of love and happiness and joy that our home felt bursting at the seams. Almost hallucinogenic, and this was before all the drugs ...

Maybe that's the difference between living and dying. Because we are all dying, every damn one of us. But if we are loving, and being loved, and FEELING, then we are living.

I am not numb. Well, parts of me are, from all the surgeries and chemo and such, but I am living this experience. It is a part of me, but not any more than all those numb parts. I am happy, and joyful and loved and I can feel ALL of that.

Love Stacy

This day will never happen again.

April 28, 2014

Dear Cancer,

Still incapacitated, I am teetering somewhere between the "peak of poison" and "pick your poison," the latter a choice of either debilitating pain or 'round-the-clock pain meds and being a total zombie. I have been in bed for five days.

Chemo on Thursday. Friday, Saturday, Sunday ... Monday. Gone. It is so weird.

I'm not stressing that I've done nothing for so long. It is, simply, what it is. But I feel like a bat. And I'm suffering from echolocation ... every time Dave's new cell phone clings, dings or rings, it sounds like some alarm going off in my house, and it's driving me crazy. He has been so patient. I am not.

I was told it would take two rounds to really understand what to expect: the first time to see what happens and the second time to know. So now I know. This will end, hopefully soon. The first time I really wasn't so sure. Anyway, I think it's dusk. Gotta go.

Love Stacy

"Sometimes the thoughts in my head get so bored they go out for a stroll through my mouth. This is rarely a good thing."

—SCOTT WESTERFELD

May 1, 2014

Dear Cancer,

This is a slow walk through hell.

For the last several days, that's all I have been thinking. This is a slow walk through hell. It's not that I'm not walking. I am. But not much. Today I feel a little better. But not much. Enough to sit down and write: *This is a slow walk through hell.*

Something is protecting me. I am not losing my mind. I may have been a bit delirious from sleeping only five of the first ninety-six hours this round. Those steroids are a bitch. But I am sane. Everything I've said is true, every emotion expressed was felt. This is a slow walk through hell.

I was so bored the other day that I picked up the careful chart I keep bedside to document my drug intake—to ensure I'm getting what I need and when—and I counted how many pills I'd ingested in the last five or so days. Fifty-two. I couldn't eat fifty-two M&Ms in that amount of time. I don't really like M&Ms, but still. That's a lot of medication.

Last night I even cried a little. I am being poisoned. I can feel it. I can taste it. I am a toxic wasteland. I felt so sick all day, my body finally purging the poltergeist inside me. I've lost seven pounds in three days. Not to worry; when I can eat, I do. And I will. It's just the nature of the beast.

But once again Dave and I had the conversation that I will not do this again. I will give it this shot. I gave it a good one eight years ago. But if this cancer comes back, forget it. If I walk through this hell and by some menacing labyrinth end up back at the gates, I am not going in.

I do not understand the insanity of our culture to absolutely fear death. We are so obsessed with prolonging life that no one seems to consider how to live it. It's not a criticism; I am grateful for the care I'm getting. I would not have chosen to give up this time. But what if this is my fate? What if cancer is what gets me? It's awful and terrible and horrible and tragic, but so are heart disease and car accidents and tornadoes. I envy those who drop dead. I hope their loved ones, who are entitled to their grief and sorrow, are at peace with the fact that their loved ones died quickly, maybe without pain and suffering.

And who the hell writes stories like Snow White? That came from somewhere. Did people really poison one another in medieval times? Were they that barbaric? And are we any different today?

It's all so crazy and it's all just words, but I will not live to die. For crying out loud, I am dying to live.

Love Stacy

Be happy while you're living, for you're a long time dead.

—SCOTTISH PROVERB

May 4, 2014

Dear Cancer,

Ten days off, ten days on. That seems to be the pattern. I am finally feeling good again.

It comes as easily as it goes; once I feel better it's hard to remember how truly awful it was. I walked into that second treatment without a worry in the world, and halfway through I could already feel it raging inside me. Forgive me, but talk about a mind fuck. Thankfully anxiety has never been a matter, cancer my only vice.

So I'm back in the saddle: went out both nights this weekend, had some fun, and laughed my ass off, however tiny it may be. And I looked good doing it.

Love Stacy

Fall seven times, stand up eight.
—JAPANESE PROVERB

May 5, 2014

Dear Cancer,

Fall seven times, stand up eight. I've done the math on this one, oh sweet little inspirational ditty. Fall seven times, stand up eight? Fall once, stand up; fall again, stand up again. Fall seven times, you need only stand up seven times after. Which funnily reminds me of my twelfth-grade calculus class, when on the last day of school the teacher called my name, announcing her student with the highest score on the final exam. *Who, me?* Stunned, I fell out of my chair.

Then, in that weird, unknowing, calculus sort of way, it clicked: maybe this *is* right. Fall seven times, stand up eight. For that is what I'm going to have to do.

This is not as easy as falling once and standing right back up. I am going to have to HEAL. Go through chemo once, get back up. Twice, get back up. Three and four times, get back up and back up again.

And then back up again.

For one is my hair. It's going to take time; who knows how long, or how it's going to look when it grows back, and how I'll like it after that. And my body, my poor, wrecked body. I am strong but it is weak. Dissected and poisoned; deadened again, when, after eight years, I was just beginning to feel some sensation. It's going to take time.

And menopause. Surgical, instantaneous, hormone thieving, hot flash inducing, bone mass reducing menopause. It is affecting me in ways unexpected, and I will have to adjust. It's going to take time.

I am worse than I was, I'll be better than I am. Worse than I was, better than I am. Worse than I was, better than I am, better than I am. Better than I am. I will fall seven times. I will stand up eight.

And I will never question my math again.

Love Stacy

What would you do if you weren't afraid?

May 6, 2014

Dear Cancer,

Today I feel great. I went to yoga, mostly to hear my teacher's voice, to listen to what she had to say, and of course, it was exactly what I needed to hear. I don't recall her words, but they worked, and there went all the cobwebs. I can't remember the last time my body felt this good.

How easy it is to forget. It is so hard to reach for peace when all you feel is pain. Honestly, I've discovered you can't grasp for joy so much as accept where you are and it will come. I have learned both times, and throughout my life, that acceptance is the answer. Not to be confused, ever, with resignation.

Life is so unfair, so complete with suffering, if we don't embrace joy there is nothing left but unfairness and suffering. If we don't learn that these are *part* of the joy, of the journey, of the beauty that makes a whole life, then we have nothing. If we don't somehow learn to be fearless, then we will be consumed by fear. I know that. I have been there.

And I am not done here. All that crap I said about not fighting this again … I know, even as I write, that I have no idea what I would do if faced with this monster once more. My travels are too many to visit the land of Coulda Woulda Shoulda. It is an empty place. Regret resides there. Worry lives there. Fear fits there. I do not. I am right here where I belong.

So as I've been told, one fire at a time. One day at a time. One step at a time. One breath at a time. Put out the fire but keep the flame.

Love Stacy

You look fine.

May 7, 2014

Dear Cancer,

Here's the thing about scarves. They have to be square. They must be lightweight. And they need to match. It's an accessory, those little extras that took me decades to learn how to wear. And now I need them every day. I have absolutely no interest in wigs.

I have taken to wearing bandanas most of the time. They are sized just right, they cover my head, I can wear them to exercise, and they are easily assembled. You should see the ritual I go through to get a scarf tied to fit. Fit to be tied is more like it.

My hair is gone now. The buzz was cute, but bald, while beautiful, just isn't pretty. I was never one to star gaze in the mirror but I notice myself frequenting them less. I don't know if the sight of myself is uncomfortable or just a reminder of this protraction. I am wishing away this year.

There is, in fact, new growth on my head. Just enough so I can feel it, but so light as not to be seen, and my scalp is definitely exposed. But it gives me hope. Maybe I'll come back as a blonde. With ambition.

Love Stacy

"Never suppress a generous thought."

—CAMILLA KIMBALL

May 10, 2014

Dear Cancer,

It's funny, the little things.

I read a disturbing article this week in *New York Magazine*[6], written by a doctor whose wife had succumbed to breast cancer. She was diagnosed at forty-three—my age—and died three years later. More striking was his demonstration, in graphic detail, of their attempt to defy the inevitable and the shocking horrors of her demise, speaking precisely to my gravest concerns. It put me in a funk for days.

So this afternoon, just hours before a formal event we attended for my daughter, I decided to treat myself to a beautiful new scarf, to accentuate a lovely new dress that's been patiently awaiting its turn. As I was leaving the boutique, an old acquaintance ran out to see me. She had

---

6   Peter B. Bach, "The Day I Started Lying to Ruth," *New York Magazine*, May 5, 2014 issue.

been reading my page, and wanted to express her support by way of sharing some scarves. And there it was: the shift. Her small gesture and great admiration brightened me right out of my darkness.

I have always been sensitive to the notion that even when life runs smoothly, our moods swing from time to time, from day to day, moment to moment. Ever wake up on the wrong side of the bed, only to be tempered by a simple call from a friend or a sweet song on the radio? Those slight changes have often helped me through, recognizing that life is never always good nor perpetually bad, but that all things come and go. For the very reason feeling happy is unsustainable, it is equally impossible to be forever down. Let it come and it will go.

We had a great night out, I have another good week ahead, and here is what I've learned on this ride. How I look is integral to how I feel. Change is both monumental and minute. Acceptance is effortless, but fear is insidious.

Let it come and it will go.

Love Stacy

"You only live once, but if you do it right, once is enough."

—MAE WEST

May 13, 2014

Dear Cancer,

Not a term I use lightly, but these hot flashes are killing me. They are so abundant and sharp, disturbing my peace during the day and destroying my rest at night. Jolted by their surge of heat, I awaken to a particular heaviness, an unfamiliar ache associated with chemo, then charged with the troubled task of returning back to sleep.

It took about three weeks after surgery to settle in, for my body to recognize that something was missing. My ovaries foremost, but all that essential estrogen that clearly kept me cool, or at least fairly regulated. I now empathize with women going through menopause, more dramatic though to be surgically shocked into it.

Interestingly, everything else has flatlined. My moods, in spite of the ups and downs of chemo, have softened. My normal day to day irritability has waned, though don't ask Dave for confirmation. It is something I can feel from within. If he is not finding me tolerable, I concede. Because if this isn't a rough patch, I don't know what is. We are routine and happy but hoping these are the worst of times. You can only really know in retrospect, and only then after you've lived your full life. And who knows when that will be.

Maybe that's why it seems like things always get better. We think our twenties are the best time of our life, only to find great joy in family or friends or career in our thirties; then seem to have figured it all out in our forties, and, I imagine, to have really done so by the next decade around.

I have always had one big wish, which I make clear all the time: I hope to be married fifty years. It's a running joke in our house that that is all I want; that David, at seventy-seven, is free to do whatever he wants and with whom, so long as we reach our golden anniversary. I wish him all the luck.

The truth is, we will never have enough time as one, but fifty years of marriage seems to cover all the bases. It ensures a long life, together, for the both of us. It gives us the opportunity to witness and enjoy our children's milestones, including the hope of seeing them fall in love and get married, and by the grace of God or whatever greatness gets us there, to be present as they bring their own children into this world.

The minute my son was born I faithfully recall the thought that I couldn't wait to be a grandmother. I had only just become a mother, but in that moment I immediately knew, in the deepest part of me, that this was what life, *my life*, was all about. Grateful for the beauty and blessings and cycle of life.

In his second-grade class book, my friend's hilarious—and obviously brilliant—son wrote, "If I could have one wish it would be to have anything I want."

Likewise, kiddo. I hope my wish comes true.

Love Stacy

Don't tell people your dreams. Show them.

May 14, 2014

Dear Cancer,

With a fleeting sense of relief I started pre-meds today. I have knocked on its door and hell is about to welcome me in. Another visit with an old friend, it will feel like no distance has passed between us. Some things may change but it will mostly be the same. And then round three will be behind me.

I have been lucky. The few events we've wanted to attend for our children happened to fall by chance on my good days. I can't help but think that graduation is right around the corner, the ceremony just days after my fourth and final treatment, when I will be mired in the depths of discomfort. My kids will attend; several of their friends are moving on. But it would have been my son had we not held him back in pre-school. I knew then it was the right decision, that he needed and we would enjoy an extra year together, but never could I have imagined what an incredible gift it would become.

The night I received my diagnosis, I was instantly grateful for the time ahead, knowing we would all be together for a normal year before Ethan leaves for college. I could see him walking that stage, and I could see myself watching the procession, with unbridled joy and pride and all the bittersweet emotion that comes with grand milestones. I promised him I would be there, feeling and looking good, with my health and my hair back.

Just one more year with the four of us under one roof. Both breaks my heart and builds it, to think of us any other way, but such is life and I am going to celebrate the hell out of it.

Love Stacy

*"Art should comfort the disturbed
and disturb the comfortable."*

—CESAR A. CRUZ

May 15, 2014

Dear Cancer,

Already just begun and I haven't even left for treatment:
the insomnia, the bloating, the endless wandering of the
mind. I could think of nothing last night but art. Not a
terrible muse, but an expensive one nonetheless. If I were
to run out and buy all the pieces I have loved, paintings
and photographs that would be lovely to live with, their
worth would not add up to one day's cost of chemotherapy.

If only I could trade it all in.

Love Stacy

"The price of anything is the amount of life you exchange for it."

—HENRY DAVID THOREAU

May 15, 2014

Dear Cancer,

There is no language profane enough for you. Chemo yes, cancer no. The former is toxic but the latter is evil. I abandon my attempt to condemn with words.

Today I learned, in addition to my prior understanding that breast cancer is often systemic, meaning it spreads easily, that although no cells may show up in the lymph nodes, the tumor develops its own blood vessels, creating an independent avenue for travel. There is no way to determine when or whether the trip has begun, until a noticeable difference in health. And by then it is too late. Metastasis is the beginning of the end. And I am worried about the spot on my back.

Chemo is applied to kill these very "seeds" that cannot be seen, and BRCA tumors respond well to a regimen of chemo plus radiation, which I am likely to undergo. At this point, bring it on.

I will be in therapy—drug rehabilitation—for a good part of the rest of my life. The idea of being medicated for decades is unsettling, yet at once reassuring, lest the shorter and terminal alternative.

This disease is so misunderstood, the worse for making its acquaintance. Chemo days really aren't so bad. There is no pain associated with the drip, just hours of patience on my behalf and boredom on Dave's. Its after effects are what really take the toll.

I surmise this good life is getting costly, but I'll pay the price if not my dues. And then I hope to owe nothing for a good long while.

Love Stacy

"Everything you want is on the other side of fear."

—JACK CANFIELD

May 15, 2014

Dear Cancer,

I know, in every cell of my being—the sick and the healthy, the dying and the developing—that fear is a sooner and more certain death than any.

I mostly live without it, and easily so. The need to perpetually persuade it away would be difficult work, but like my marriage, neither effort has been my challenge. For which I am both fortunate and grateful.

But I must, too, accept the improbable as a possibility; to live cautiously without expectation, to live freely without consumption, and to live fiercely with the unknown. It is a very delicate balance.

I have but one chance to make my mark, to leave a legacy of love to my children. A force to endure their lifetime, not any time soon, but at long, long last.

Love Stacy

"Be strong when you are weak. Be brave when you are scared. Be humble when you are victorious."

—MICHELLE MOSCHETTI

May 16, 2014

Dear Cancer,

Despite the many bathroom breaks to release Cytoxan, toxic to the bladder, the Adriamycin coming out, just as it goes in—Kool-Aid red, the routine hand washing to avoid contamination for everyone around me, the bloating and nausea from Taxotere kept largely at bay by Aloxi and Emend, as well as the dexamethasone steroid which I was granted permission to stop taking after three doses instead of the usual six due to its vicious insomniac effect, I slept not through but for some of the night. Little victories.

Today Neulasta, tomorrow the battle against bone pain; Claritin, Motrin and Vicodin required. Senokot and pro-biotics for my belly. Zofran and Phenergan as needed, but won't be. A double 07 of drugs. With a cocktail that sexy, watch out Bond, here I come.

Disarming the enemy one conquest at a time, and fighting the good fight.

Like a girl. And a motherfucker.

Love Stacy

*"What seems to us as bitter trials
are often blessings in disguise."*
—OSCAR WILDE

May 18, 2014

Dear Cancer,

Weekends are killing time after Thursday infusions, a double entendre of demise. Clearly the chemo is doing its job, cells dying off everywhere, exhausting every bit of my being. And there is nothing, absolutely nothing to do or be done, but to endure. No waiting for time to pass, but to pass, painfully, through time.

Today I got out of bed for a while, feeling somewhat productive. It is forced, the getting up and doing, but I was able to dress, do a bit of laundry, watch the end of a movie, and two hours later, trudge achingly back to bed. It had felt like an entire afternoon. The worst part—though how to measure misery—is the absolute failure of digestion and total distortion of taste. The factory is on strike. So much as sipping water is strained. Eating anything is the opposite of pleasure, and all of this to the extreme.

Muddling through the mess, I have another week of discomfort, hopefully moderate; made somewhat more tolerable for knowing, after this, there's only one more stretch.

Love Stacy

Once in a while, blow your own damn mind.

May 20, 2014

Dear Cancer,

Sunday I was so sick. Monday, a little better, but still terribly fatigued. Chemo sucks. It feels like an animal crawled inside my mouth and died. Instead, one crawled in my pool and died, and I spotted it just as I was about to force myself to eat lunch. Honestly, I would have preferred throwing up to sitting around not throwing up, that is how awful chemo is.

Dave took care of it and claimed, "I got him!" proud of his persistence, and patience with me. And then we laughed, together and aloud. We can't wait for our life to not suck.

But oh, it made me sick. And then, I was sick again. Of myself.

All the complaining, the explaining, the suffering and sharing. I could articulate its aspects, describe each discomfort, disprove every myth about this rotten remedy. I can't help it, and hopefully it helps; to dissolve, not diminish, the dismay. I had no idea what I was getting into. No one does. But enough already. It's making me sick.

Then today, I woke up feeling great. Good enough to go to yoga, a full week earlier than last time. Steamed through class, surprised myself, determined to make it through. Of all the things I could have blown, it was my own damn mind. Pushing and breathing and thinking, *I am not going down.*

I am not going down.

I am not going down without a fight.

Love Stacy

"Life begins at the end of your comfort zone."

—NEALE DONALD WALSCH

May 22, 2014

Dear Cancer,

I just discovered the most wonderful thing. We have in our backyard a trampoline that, call me a kid, I enjoy on occasion. It's really fun, and fabulous exercise, but bothered my hair, always too fine to stay tied. But today, on whatever impulse, I climbed up and realized I can jump bald, no tangles, no trouble. It was oddly exciting. Welcome to my world of tiny triumphs.

The afternoon of my diagnosis, I was sitting on my daughter's bed, four days before her sixteenth birthday, shopping with her online for a few pre-celebration gifts. It was a sweet and rare occasion, afternoons usually reserved for homework and unwinding, alone, as teenagers do. The phone rang, and not a moment into the call, I ran out and began pacing the house, alarmed with disbelief. When I returned to her room, I handed her the credit card, asked her to finish the transaction herself and we embraced. I hugged her and swayed and cried, and told her I had cancer. That things were going to get bad before they get better. And when I let her go, she was crying, too.

To be expected, perhaps, but my daughter, my sweet, beautiful, baby girl, is tough as nails. She may bend, but only when hammered and, believe me, someone's thumb has been smashed in the wake. I can count on my hands the times I've seen her cry in sixteen years, and most include serious injury and false or unfair accusation of wrongdoing. Much of my strength comes from observing her, and maybe hers comes from me, but she has the gift of not getting hurt, and it is an awe to behold.

When she came home from school the next day and told me she was going to donate her hair, I thought her valiant but didn't realize what she meant: she wanted to give it to me. It was the most compassionate moment we have ever shared, and I will forever be proud.

Then I resolved to forego a wig, and she decided to hang on. Down to her waist, she has the most magnificent mane, and I am not speaking through the filtered eyes of her mother but through the hard lens of truth. Her hair is absolutely gorgeous. But yesterday she voluntarily had it cut, to donate to Locks of Love, an organization that provides hairpieces to children with long-term medical hair loss.

She wasn't happy. Her tress was difficult to part with, shocking to be fair, after so many years of growth. We left her alone for a while, and after dinner she came back down, holding the braid up to the blunt cut of her hair, shooting selfies and joking around. It takes time to adjust to change, to sacrifice, however inconsequential that may be.

I couldn't help but wonder if, in her teen-spirited grief, she has thought of me, of what it is like to surrender, to suffer, and to survive. Surely a rich lesson has been learned.

Because, really, I can shower in minutes and jump without fuss, but show me a woman who, by leaps and bounds, would rather be bald than have a bad hair day.

Love Stacy

My body's an atrocity
an absurdity at best
these giant things upon me
feel like snow globes on my chest

I could run and jump and spin around
and stand upon my head
they won't move or even jiggle
for they're just as hard as lead

I know this pain and process
are only temporary
and so I joke and laugh it off
and continue to be merry

JANUARY 5, 2006

"Do not regret growing older. It is a privilege denied to many."

—AUTHOR UNKNOWN

May 27, 2014

Dear Cancer,

If there is one event that most altered my life, that gave me the perspective I possess today, it was not the excitement of my wedding day or the blessed birth of my two children, or even my first diagnosis, though this second one is re-forming me once again. It was the morning, when I was just twenty-five and she twenty-six, that we awoke to learn of the sudden death of David's sister Angela.

She was, by all accounts, one of my dearest friends, and my biggest fan. When I told her that David and I were getting married—finally—she cried for joy. Our friendship, which took form in never-ending talks on our drives together to Austin and back, on long walks and in ice cream shops, healed the troubled relationship she had with David when he and I first met. And her death forever changed me.

For one, it seemed to seal our marriage in a way I can't quite articulate. We had only been married for seven months and suddenly we were bound by her death; by the unimaginable loss, at such a young age for all of us. We visited her at the funeral home, a viewing I needed for closure. We discussed and supported our parents' choice to buy a large family plot, where we could all be buried. That in itself has always provided me with a sense of permanency, and peace. At twenty-five, I already had my final resting place.

It all sounds so grave, but Dave and I speak of these things often. Especially now. That we will be buried there together, no matter what happens. That life can get complicated. If I should perish early, he could be married again, perhaps longer than we would be together. And who goes where then?

The other day we were driving home and we spotted a bright red Corvette. I have never been a fan, but Dave is, and he said if I ever wanted to surprise him, he would like it in yellow. Not happening. So then he said he should just get one now, because if I died then it would really seem like a mid-life crisis car. We were cracking up. Amidst all this heavy stuff, that is how we relate. I told him it was worse for me to think he'd buy that stupid car than to be with another woman.

That is the blessing of Angela's death. We take absolutely nothing for granted. We never part without knowing it could be the last time. We love openly and laugh as much as possible and we don't take things too seriously except for the serious things, which we face head on. No subject is off the table. We are not afraid to speak the truth, all our truths. We talk about *everything*.

And we miss her. Today would have been her forty-fifth birthday. I can still hear her voice. I remember our conversations. I feel her spirit. And I can't wait to see her again. But it's going to be a while.

Love Stacy

*"Don't feel sorry for yourself.
Only assholes do that."*

—HARUKI MURAKAMI

May 29, 2014

Dear Cancer,

Well, I just found out I will have seven weeks of radiation
this summer. Twenty-five rounds on my boob, for that's
really all it is: skin, implant and fucking cancer. Then eight
rounds of more intensive radiation—a boost—at the site of
the excision, where the tumor was removed. My radiologist
was so sweet and compassionate and started by saying he
already knew me, from attending the Tumor Board meeting
at which dozens of doctors studied and made recommen-
dations concerning my case. I am in good hands.

And then he said that rare, alluring word: that his objec-
tive, their goal, is to "cure" me. They are trying to save
my life; striving for a long life because I am so young. So
young. I kept hearing *so young*. That the tumor was very

aggressive, and is often so in young women, so it needs to be treated aggressively.

We carefully went over my pathology report which, as always, was terrifying, with a dose of good news as well. And I am okay with this. He said radiation will be easy compared to chemo, and the side effects don't sound too terrible, though of course there are consequences. Discoloration, skin burn, fatigue, and a bit of radiation to my lung and esophagus. No deodorant, no swimming, never mind being land locked here all summer, in the heat, which normally doesn't bother me but is a deadly combination with all these damn hot flashes.

Last night I awoke to not one but three in a row. It feels like catching fire. Unable to fall back asleep, instead I began to feel something I hadn't quite yet experienced. A bit of sadness, maybe, some frustration, though dare not self-pity. I absolutely refuse to feel sorry for myself.

Except that we are talking about my health, and more importantly, my life, and the quality of those years ahead. And for once, I am entitled to feel upset about it, if only for half a night.

I have made the decision to turn these next few months into a stay-cation, starting a list of all the things I want to do here in town this summer. Restaurants we've wanted to try but never get around to, creatures of habit always returning to our favorite spots; art spaces and museums I seem to miss but every year or so; maybe end up at a spa sometime.

Treat every day, even in treatment, as equal, because each day is the only one I get.

Love Stacy

"Courage, dear heart."

—C. S. LEWIS

June 1, 2014

Dear Cancer,

Funk funk funk funk

funk funk funk funk

funk funk funk funk

fuck.

Love Stacy

"Believe you can and you're halfway there."

—THEODORE ROOSEVELT

June 1, 2014

Dear Cancer,

My dad and his wife came in town this weekend from Florida to see me. I knew in the beginning he did not grasp the gravity of the situation. And now I'm thinking, neither did I. Maybe from visiting with him and discussing the details, or perhaps what I learned from our two-hour consultation with the radiologist, the more I understand my pathology, the more reality bites.

I'm not sure if my family of doctors just isn't saying so or if they truly have faith. Statistically, my prognosis is grim.

All this courage and bravery and fearlessness, for what it's worth, has served me well. In the wake of surgery after surgery, chemotherapy and all its horrors, soon thirty-three rounds of radiation and then a decade of endocrine therapy, I have kept my head on straight.

But now it is setting in. A rigor mortis of fear.

I made it to yoga class yesterday. Lying on the floor in resting pose, I turned my head to the right and there it was, on my water bottle, staring me straight in the face. Expiration date: May 03 2016.

Damn the prophecy, and all that fucking plastic is going to outlast every one of us anyway. But I am scared.

The weight of suffering hasn't brought me to my knees; it has made me stronger. I can carry that around all day long, because when it's done, it's done. The physical pain over, it is behind me, and no longer matters.

But the burden remains. Waging war against recurrence, my doctors are trying everything, but there is no crystal ball and no guarantee. Saddled with the unknown, letting it out lightens the load.

And so I must go now, pull myself out, grip by grip from the deep abyss, and back up to the mountaintop. Step by step.

Love Stacy

"If there is light it will find you."

—CHARLES BUKOWSKI

June 3, 2014

Dear Cancer,

Last day of school and my kids are thrilled. But it feels like half a year without a trace.

My only evidence, the mass I noticed the first week in January, while away on vacation over winter break. Doctor's appointment in January; MRI early February; surgery late February; diagnosis early March.

And then all hell broke loose. Now I understand the true meaning of that expression: free rocks falling, avalanche upon avalanche of testing and treatment, suffering and pain, comprehension and concern, all closing in on us, suffocating our world.

It's been three months now, on a very rocky road. Certainly I was bound to trip at some point.

Slowly but surely, I am scraping myself back up. If not yet into the light, then definitely into the heat. While walking our dogs this evening, wearing a knit turban instead of my usual bandana, my head was so hot I had to take the damn thing off.

Just the other day as we were leaving the house, Dave asked if I was going to get a hat. I had completely forgotten to cover my head. I rarely do in my house, but I have yet to bare myself in public, or with anyone beside my kids. It's a curious thing; we are not modest here. Dave and I are comfortable in our own skin and always wanted our children to be. It's not like we prance around nude, but neither is anyone expected to be dressed when comfortably at home. And yet, my bald head makes me feel naked in some way. A private part of me exposed.

But I am starting to get over it. The more I know, the less everything else matters. I want one thing, and that is to live. Vanity aside, future ahead.

We have, together, so much to live for, and my children especially have not lived long enough with us. A forced layer of independence thrust upon them, they have been truly loving and incredibly strong. But for all the years of immense joy and happiness and laughter, those sweet memories of early and middle childhood, they will remember mostly these high school years, now marred by my disease. I do not want to burden them with dread.

Summer is our favorite time, and it's time to embrace the season.

With brightness and lightness and light.

Love Stacy

"You gain strength, courage and confidence by every experience in which you really stop to look fear in the face."

—ELEANOR ROOSEVELT

June 4, 2014

Dear Cancer,

Out of the funk and into the fray: pre-meds start today. My fourth and final round of chemo, and I never thought I'd say it, but I hope it's enough. I was grateful when told I would only undergo four rounds, optimistic that meant things were not so bad. And after the first two, I thought I'd never be able to endure more than my fair share.

But when the fear crept in, I finally realized this is not about the damage, or pain, or chronic discomfort in my body. It is, truly, about saving my life. Everything, every single experience I must confront, is secondary, irrelevant, even trivial compared to survival. I am willing to suffer any consequence to stay alive. To knock this out, once, twice and for all.

In the funk I felt the shift. The striving we all hope for, to live purely in the moment, with appreciation, clarity and kindness. I find myself being more loving and less bothered by the little things that make up our daily lives, with busy children and a spouse at home. I am so lucky. It's a lot of togetherness, and it began to wear on us this last round. Until, besieged by fear, I realized instead I am surrounded by love.

We are more compassionate with each other, Dave and me, and he is even more determined to move forward, continue with our many plans, most of them dreams for his retirement which we have yet to celebrate. A rehabilitation from the paralysis of dread.

Crying for days, I was totally, emotionally and physically exhausted. It's an impossible way to live. I had no choice but to bounce back, pull through, reclaim the positive and recapture the light.

I do not know how long I have to live. It scares me to even say that. With the weighted mystery of the unknown, I wondered if every move I make is now in vain, or if each and every moment counts. And so the great conundrum: do I live like I'm dying or survive like I won't?

Love Stacy

Think like a proton and stay positive.

June 5, 2014

Dear Cancer,

Dave and I talk routinely, not altogether jokingly, about which one of us will outlive the other. We laughingly construct fantasies of dying together. Not because we would ever take our own lives, but because we never want to be taken from each other. These days we are convinced that even if it's many years from now, I am going first.

Almost preachingly, I have said before that none of us knows when our time will come. A little something that helps keep me sane. The impossible prediction of our death is the truest, hardest fact of life. The difference for me is that I have a known risk, a serious and measurable threat to my mortality. To compare it to any other hardship is brazenly unfair.

Not a betrayal of love, nor the loss of a job, bankruptcy, or a building burned. All things painful, irrevocable even, but with perseverance can be overcome; with hard work, emotional strength, the essential grit of accepting responsibility. The very same efforts I have put forth. Mind over matter. Except this is the stuff of science, and wildly beyond my control.

This is my truth, our reality, not a metaphorical look in the mirror but a daily illumination of our life. Developed in darkness, but bravely seen through the light.

We do not throw pity parties around here. And I am not having one now. Dave has already made clear he is serving champagne at our funerals, even if he's not the one bartending. We have a lot of celebrating to do before then, but stick around. They are going to be fun.

Love Stacy

"It always seems impossible until it's done."

—NELSON MANDELA

June 5, 2014

Dear Cancer,

I finished my last chemotherapy treatment today. This doesn't mean it's over. I have to get through the side effects and each round is measured in three week intervals, not complete until blood counts stop fluctuating and return to normal. But no more sitting through.

I was asked to read a poem[7] aloud and ring the bell while the entire staff cheered *Hooray!* and I'm not sure why, since I still have radiation and really, interminable treatment ahead, but I cried. Maybe because my beautiful children were standing by my side, joining me on this last day, and I realized how important it was for them to see what I've been going through. Not to torment them but to expose them to the very adversity that makes us all stronger.

7   Signaling the conclusion of chemotherapy and radiation treatment, it has become a widespread tradition at many cancer centers for patients to ring a bell after reading the poem *Ringing Out* by Irve Le Moyne.

I used to wonder where they would get it, growing up in a peaceful, loving home, in stark contrast to my own. Until one day I had a conversation, after my first diagnosis when my children were still quite young, with a woman who had lost her teenage daughter to sudden death, and I expressed this very concern. She reminded me that difficult times will come, in what form we do not know, but not to waste my time wishing. Hardship awaits.

We are graced with such prosperity, so maybe here it is: our family's great misfortune. Something is stirring inside them. I hope it is not worry or fear, but eternal love and growing strength, simply from watching me endure. And it is enough.

It is all enough.

Love Stacy

Keep calm and kick cancer's ass.

June 6, 2014

Dear Cancer,

Miserable. I am so swollen and bloated from yesterday's infusion, all those nasty fluids trapped inside me, spending a mostly sleepless night both in a deep chill and layered in sweat, my head on fire from hot flash after hot flash after hot flash.

But it is the last time—I hope, I think, I pray. My oncologist is out of the country for the next two weeks and I want to consult with her one last time before having the port removed. This miserable, painful, ugly, burning, stinging, swollen port surgically removed from my chest. I want to be sure—reassured—once and for all, that these four treatments are going to be enough.

Not that anyone can truly predict the outcome, but after last week's fall into the deep abyss of doom, I need a boost of confidence and in her I have faith. So I will wait for her return, and a final, lasting decision to be made.

I will spend today forcing down fluids, making our trip back to the cancer center for my last Neulasta shot. I hope, I think, I pray.

And then on with it. Waiting out the next ten days of symptoms and side effects and hopefully the end of this part of the journey.

Love Stacy

Gynecologist
Radiologist
Surgical Radiologist
to name a few

then to Pathologist
onto Oncologist
Anesthesiologist
General Surgeon and Plastics ensue

back to Pathologist
meet with Oncologist
and now Dermatologist
for my skin's suffered, too

screenings for breast cancer
then for ovarian
a check of my skin to be safe

blood work for gene testing
pre-op and post-op
and pregnancy just to be
sure since I'm late

bandages changing, drains need removal
expansions come every two weeks
not quite a lab rat
or pretty pin cushion
but one day I'll say
it's enough

to get through these horrors
and frequent appointments
you have to stay strong and be tough

JANUARY 16, 2006

"Open your mouth only if what you are going to say is more beautiful than silence."

—AUTHOR UNKNOWN

June 6, 2014

Dear Cancer,

Every fucking Friday after chemo, my computer fails me in some way. It is the one thing I know I will outlast.

A dear friend of mine came in town this week to be with me yesterday. We share a wonderfully storied past; her husband was my first true love. My relationship with him ended in dramatic fashion, just as it had carried on, and I met David six weeks later. So, yeah, my marriage is my rebound. But it works, and so does our beautiful friendship. I am deeply grateful for so much lasting love in my life.

Last night when she joined us for dinner, we got to talking about mediums, and connections, a look into our pasts, acute facts of our lives never revealed to anyone, yet, in her experience, others seemed to know.

My daughter wasn't buying it. She is ever the realist. But I also know that she just hasn't evolved yet, into the understanding that while fortune tellers might be bullshit, we are all spiritually connected. Intertwined forever, and that even beyond our physical existence, love will endure.

It is my only legacy to leave behind, whenever that may be. And I am confident, when the time comes, she will know it. She will recognize it, and feel it, and believe that I've been there with her all along.

Love Stacy

Don't let anyone with bad eyebrows tell you shit about life.

June 10, 2014

Dear Cancer,

I am finally emerging from the wicked weekend, wretched and rotten and wrong. Taste is still torture. I am tormented by stench. Everything, everything stinks. I would exchange my good sense to never smell anything, ever again. And all I could say, or think, or feel, was *I'd rather be dead than feel like this.*

I am not good at being miserable. A dreadful fate, worse than death. And then I got it all figured out. Chemo, you little shit. You're supposed to help by killing off cancer, but instead you prepare us for if you can't. Making it easier to understand my choices, so I won't be disappointed in the end. Because I'd rather be dead than feel like this.

Cancer, no doubt, is trying to outsmart me. Charged with the task of chasing me down. I can flee or I can fight, but

I cannot win. There is no escape from its threat. Because there is no cure.

A friend of mine recently pondered my thoughts on spray tans. I know little but she knows less about the ridiculous ways in which we can buy back our vanities. It's not that I don't care; I have said before that I want to look good because it makes me feel the same. I simply believe in doing the best we can with what we've got. Spraying and paying for sun seems a highlight of what is wrong with our society.

I know I have been jaded. I will never view life the same way again. Instead of noticing the number of wrinkles, imagine your days may be numbered. For there lies my reflection. This is what I face, every single day, for the rest of my life.

I am as pale as a ghost right now, though my fine lines and sun spots have miraculously disappeared. One of the hidden gems of chemo: beauty's best kept secret! And I've been lucky. I still have most of my eyelashes and brows, admittedly, something I had hoped would be spared. One less thing to make me look sick.

But I can honestly say that even if I'd lost them all, if my fingernails had fallen off, which could have happened, too, I would have been okay. And I wouldn't get a spray tan.

Love Stacy

"Sometimes the people around you won't understand your journey. They don't need to, it's not for them."

—JOUBERT BOTHA

June 12, 2014

Dear Cancer,

The other day I received a disturbing message from a distant relative, already presuming me dead and therefore encouraging me—holding me responsible, actually—to repair the difficult relationship I share with my mother. And not for my sake, but for my mother's. I am often addressed with misunderstanding, but this was arrogant and insensitive. Well intentioned perhaps, but terribly ill-conceived.

For one, and let me be clear: I am not dying, but living with hope. And though my mother and I have always struggled, since the very beginning of time, things happen to be as good as I could hope for right now. We try our best. It is all I ask and the most I can give.

And so I got to thinking about reconciliation and redemption and how not every story has a perfect ending.

Except that mine does, and will, because no matter the circumstance, or the timing, or the order in which we go, I have done right by my children. Every decision I have ever made has been in their best interest, and though I haven't been perfect, for no one is, I have chosen and created and lived—with devotion, conviction and might—a life with my family filled with harmony and guidance, unconditional understanding and respect, and deep, profound love.

Whenever I think of friends who have lost their beloved parents, or those with the living who have loving, fulfilling adult relationships with them now, I never look to my past with envy or resentment but instead to my present with pride. To the family I have been so lucky to call my own. David, and my two children. They are my everything; and everything now, compared to my upbringing, has changed. No grip on the past, I live for my future. I have broken the cycle; of disconnection, anger, hysteria and humiliation. That, I have reconciled. And this life, *my* life, is my redemption.

Dave and I have been together now twenty-four years this month, longer than I lived in my childhood home. An old friend of mine, inadvertently responsible for our meeting and nearly as distant as my mentioned kin, redeemed me with her beautiful words, that "the true worth and essence of any relationship has little to do with where we come from, and everything to do with who we are."

For the first time in months, I went today for a mani-pedi, not quite out of the woods for risk of infection, but enough. I overheard some women talking about a celebrity; whom he is dating and why he is attracted to her, and what on earth this particular woman sees in him. And I thought, *How incredibly strange?* That anyone thinks they know anything about people with whom they do not share their lives is, quite simply, ludicrous.

Many people come into our lives, by family, in friendship, or otherwise. Those who stay are there for good reason, and those who don't maybe gone with fair measure. I shall not base my fate on the feelings of others, nor do I live so they may not suffer.

But make no mistake. I am going to survive. In life and in love, for now and eternity, and only for those who matter.

Love Stacy

"I have decided to be happy because it is good for my health."

—VOLTAIRE

June 17, 2014

Dear Cancer,

Coming out from under my cloud, we had a fantastic weekend spent with favorite friends who were in town visiting. Me. Visiting *me*. Which felt so good. We shared several meals, hysterical laughter and general fun times, and I am finding that is the most important, if not the only thing, moving me along. Living life and having fun. I absolutely have to get out of my head.

My doctor confirmed today there is no other way to live. That certain factors, combined with appropriate treatment, are in my favor. And to believe, simply and firmly, this is not coming back.

My son has recently been checking in with me, "Are you

okay, Mom?" Probably noticing some sadness settling in. That, or I have a bitchy resting face.

But I'm getting past it, back into life, and even though confronting radiation just ahead, I have to keep busy and therefore happy.

I am still in pain, but it's from this damn port which comes out tomorrow, so I should be on the mend soon.

And I can live with a little pain. But I cannot live at all without laughter.

Love Stacy

"In victory, you deserve champagne; in defeat, you need it."

—NAPOLEON BONAPARTE

June 18, 2014

Dear Cancer,

Port is OUT. Stings like a bitch and was infected with cellulitis but no one seemed too bothered by that but me. Ten days of antibiotics and changing the dressing and I should be fine, leaving me with exactly one day of "nothing" before starting radiation. That particular date happens to be the anniversary of my meeting Dave, so it will have to begin with mimosas and end with champagne.

Mentally I am feeling better. Because there really is no choice but to live like there is nothing to worry about, lest I waste whatever days I have left, which hopefully amount to many years. The thought of anything less is just too burdensome to carry, and so has been cast aside. If this means feigning ignorance, so be it. Still wise with vigilance, oh, cancer the wicked.

Honestly, I'm not quite sure how I am holding up,

considering the circumstances. My life is like a horror film, if ever there was one. Scarred and scored for radiation, blue lines and tape covering my chest and sides; a bullseye left, right and center. Today marked my fourth surgery in four months. And though I have claimed to know what hell feels like, now I know how it appears: as the innards of a hospital.

Awaiting my procedure this morning, Dave and I were taking it all in: patients, many hairless like me, lined up on gurneys, tubes and wires and all manner of machines attached to our wasting bodies with no privacy at all, not that I cared. The land of the sick. I looked at Dave, gestured something about how awful this all was, and for some reason we both started cracking up. Really, this is our life?

So depressing it was laughable.

I refuse to identify with the ill. I am healthy. And young, and strong. I have always taken good, no, great care of myself. And I will continue. It's called, to me, self-respect. If there is any injustice in this tragedy—the crisis of illness—it is to have to own this disease, denying me everything I have worked for, and all that I need: my good health.

The great balancing act of living with malady. And the bonfire of vanity.

Love Stacy

"There will come a time when you believe everything is finished. That will be the beginning."

—LOUIS L'AMOUR

June 22, 2014

Dear Cancer,

Day eighty-one of chemo and I should be feeling better. But I'm not. Three more days to go, officially, and my four rounds will be complete, but I am still suffering from the port/surgery/infection, and I feel pretty beaten down. And then in a week I start thirty-three rounds of radiation which surely isn't going to help any.

People often ask me how I write and from where it comes. I don't even know what to call this. It feels like screaming to me.

I know there will be an end to this treatment. But not really. I'm soon to get a drug semi-annually to promote bone growth since I am now at risk for osteoporosis, due to early menopause, which has dreadful and frightening side effects including suppressed immune system. Then the endocrine therapy for a minimum of ten years which, I am told by my doctor, is going to be really awful for the first six months—hot flashes, bone pain. Not to be confused, of course, with other "normal" aches, plus my already altered state of being So. Fucking. Hot. All. The. Time. And then I should get used to it.

When am I going to get used to this? I feel like my body is being destroyed. Ruined to save me. Suffer the consequences in order to live, or live without them and die. Those are my alternatives. And they suck.

Seven weeks of radiation, followed by a month of fatigue, a hardened implant and surgery for reconstruction, and I am so, so tired of feeling bad. Maybe I'm just scared, and I have to get through this next phase like everything else. Day eleven of chemo and I thought I'd never make it.

But here I am, seventy days later—ten weeks have passed since that sorry day—and only eight weeks ahead before I ring the next bell.

That is when I was told to start counting as a survivor. Again.

And I am waiting, wanting, ready to begin.

Love Stacy

No where to go
My body is caged
Mind swollen inside my head
I can move
But only from this side to that
The small space in between

No room for sleep
I toss and I turn
Saving by day my exhaustion
Storing it up for the prayer of peace,
Quiet body, restful mind

But it all comes out at night
This visit, these thoughts
I don't need this shit

My body is trapped
Scars staring me in the face
In my way
Only the one but it shows

I am ready
For rest, for my life and for sleep
Freedom from this wreck of my body
and heavy state of mind

Let me out of these walls
I am living within
I can walk, even run
I ponder and pray
I am ready
and need to be done

JANUARY 27, 2006

*"Be in love with your life,
every minute of it."*

—JACK KEROUAC

June 29, 2014

Dear Cancer,

Still bandaged and bruised, today is my first and only day free from treatment and without drugs in over four months. I am still not one hundred percent, afraid I may never feel like my old self again.

Just four days between the end of chemo and the start of radiation, and if I didn't get out of town, out of my house, and out of my head, I might have lost my mind.

So we went to New York. A feast for the soul, it is my favorite place on earth.

Last minute, spur of the moment and totally spontaneous, we have friends and family there but it was not about them. No calls, no visits, and no apologies. This trip was for me, and us, and nobody else. It was the first time I have felt joy in a very long time.

Some peace as well, though a different story. Every moment was exhilarating. But for all our excitement, I would wish for more. Such is travel. And experience. And fun. I want to do so much in this life.

Not only to get back to New York, and not just to see the world. But ever more specifically: to live a whole life. To visit the future of my children, thus the future for me. To get to experience everything I want to do. Everything I hope for. And everything I deserve. I am greedy with desire.

On Broadway we saw *Hedwig and the Angry Inch* with Neil Patrick Harris. The show was amazing. He was brilliant. It was extraordinary entertainment. And as Hedwig shed her wigs, I let something go, too; relating with outrage, feeling as much a freak as she.

We went to Brooklyn to see the Kara Walker exhibit, but the line was over a mile long and by the time we walked to the end of it, I was soaked from the heat and the drugs and the trek, and I would have passed out from the wait so we left. No time to spare and no chance to get back.

We walked the perimeter of Central Park, spent time in

Soho, West Village and wanted to hit the Whitney but ran out of time. And I missed the Jennifer Aniston sighting by only one day.

Dear Cancer, we were on a break.

As I looked around at all the people, many of them staring at me, it felt like everyone, in all manner of condition, was luckier in health than me. The unafflicted. And the free.

We are so fortunate to have the freedom to travel, the privilege to experience all this rich life has to offer, and yet we are enslaved by my disease.

Maybe I want more than the average, and the ordinary. I do not know how many years are left, how many places I will get to go, and take my children; how many more opportunities we will have to travel together. So many sights I want to see and things I want to do. And I don't know if it can wait.

This excursion was exactly what I needed. We had the time of our lives. We laughed and we loved and were together and alone. I was so grateful for the change of scenery, a break from our everyday hell. But it was also a reminder of all things ahead. My life, my future. Everything feels urgent, yet nothing can be rushed.

I have to live every single moment to its fullest. And then just wait and see.

Love Stacy

"Experience: the most brutal of teachers. But you learn, my God do you learn."
—C. S. LEWIS

July 1, 2014

Dear Cancer,

Countdown starts ... now.

Radiation began yesterday but instead of my first treatment they scanned me again, in order to be perfectly aligned with my initial simulation. Repeated each week, proper positioning must be ensured within a two-millimeter window. No margin of error. If only eradicating cancer could be so precise.

Lying on the board, panels circulating my body, I felt like I was on the set of *Star Wars*, at once fascinated and frightened. My life, in science non-fiction.

Scan. Pivot right, machines rotate and scan. Return, pivot

left, rotate and repeat. Lights on, lights off, and quickly back on again. Two large monitors flickering numbers and notes, pertinent information. My name illuminated on the upper left corner of right screen and lower right corner of left screen.

Backlit panels of hirsute sky, bright and deeply blue, scattered with clouds and a touch of flowering branches, shine down from the ceiling in an obvious effort to keep the calm. Peering above into the false open air, I wish for my stars to realign; to rid me of any and imminent peril.

Scan, pivot, rotate, radiate. Lights off, lights on. Repeat.

This process is deceiving, the stealth of these machines, truly amazing. Silent, painless and without warning, I lie in wait, unaware of signs of danger though its target is my body. Its secret, my future.

And the best quote from *Star Wars*?

"Never tell me the odds."[8]

Love Stacy

---

8   *Star Wars: Episode V - The Empire Strikes Back*, directed by Irvin Kershner (Lucasfilm, 1980).

"If you live to be a hundred, I hope I live to be a hundred minus one day so I never have to live without you." —Winnie the Pooh

—JOAN POWERS, INSPIRED BY A.A. MILNE

July 6, 2014

Dear Cancer,

One week from today, my maternal grandmother will be ninety-seven years old. I called her yesterday. She said I sound great; she sounds amazing. She is. At ninety-six, she still lives at home, alone. She works and drives and has good physical and mental health. There is no reason she won't live to see one hundred, and I'm not even halfway. There is such longevity in my family; and irony. Why did I get this fucking disease?

One in eight. We hear it all the time. One in eight women will be diagnosed with breast cancer. But that is no longer my truth.

A few weeks ago, one of my dearest friends—our very closest couple—was diagnosed with breast cancer. It was not my place to say who or what, when or where. But why??? Not one in eight. Now a quarter of us, of the closest to me. I am so angry with this disease.

Why are so many young women being diagnosed? It's almost like we are catching it; so prevalent to seem contagious. Some believe it is because women are being diagnosed earlier. Some truth, to be sure. But I call bullshit. I was thirty-five at first blush, and only forty-three the second time around, which now I know had been developing for years.

We are in the prime of our lives. And much too young to succumb to disease.

For the past week I have been exercising daily, and in the last five days feeling really good. But I have been burdened with my friend's news; hurting for the journey on which she has embarked. It is a difficult road, and lonely; and I have felt selfish on my path. Our plight and plea the same, this is no longer only about me.

But I am also heavy with hope. I have always believed I would live a long life; that I would get to enjoy for many, many years my marriage, our children, and our very special friends. There is no way this disease can take that from me. Nor from her. And not from us.

First as friends and now with foe, somehow we ended up in the same boat. But we shall sail through life in the company of each other, growing old together, and wise.

Tomorrow I turn forty-four. But today I pray.

Love Stacy

She loved life and it loved her right back.

July 7, 2014

Dear Cancer,

Today is my birthday. Seven-seven-seventy. I've said it a million times. For every treatment, test, surgery, procedure, infusion, injection and blood draw, I have to identify myself. State your name and birthdate: Stacy Middleman. Seven-seven-seventy. You can guess my lucky number.

But I don't feel lucky today. In the last few months, my body has aged fifteen years. I can only hope to catch up to it. Starting now, I have radiation five days a week for six more weeks. I get my bone booster this week, an injection twice a year, every year. When radiation completes, I begin endocrine therapy, for ten years, minimum. Three thousand six hundred and fifty pills. I can only hope to catch each one.

Doc said this is the most critical part of prevention. She said no matter how awful I feel, I must stick with it. Bone pain, hot flashes, vaginal atrophy. No pills, no patch, no soy. Absolutely no estrogen. Anything with comfort could kill me.

I have been offered anti-depressants. Studies show a low dose can combat the hot flashes, and I am beginning to understand the science. But I refuse. I am not depressed. And I don't want any more meds in my system.

I am not a girl with issues. Just a woman, interrupted.

Fourteen years ago we took our first vacation together as a family, to Club Med in Florida. And there it was, the discovery of my first, and only, anxiety: I was afraid of heights. I was climbing a three-story ladder to attempt trapeze, one of the celebrated activities at this resort. Way up high in the open air, stomach aflutter, I fearfully grabbed hold, swinging and screaming profanities the whole way down. It was a family club, and I was warned. I couldn't help myself.

It makes me laugh to think of it. I remember so much from that trip. Yoga on the beach, reading Sedaris by the pool. Forcing naps in the afternoon. The kids, so darn cute, at only two and three years old, participating in the evening performances. The face paint and the food, and celebrating Ethan's fourth birthday. In three weeks, he will be eighteen.

For all the joys I have to look back on, I must look ahead

just as far. I have raised a child into an adult. He is still my baby and barely a young man. I want to escort him into mature adulthood, down the aisle, and beyond. Dave may be retired, but I am not. My work is not done.

Tonight we will celebrate together, just the four of us. It is the first time in ten years my children have been with me on my birthday, after a decade of sleepaway camp and travels. Perhaps it is no coincidence they are home this year. I feel lucky today.

At forty-four, I have half a life—and entire lifetime—in front of me. I have to take it day by day, but I want to count in years.

Love Stacy

"Do what is right, not what is easy."

—ROY T. BENNETT (ABRIDGED)

July 11, 2014

Dear Cancer,

I think my follicles may be percolating. My scalp, usually smooth to the touch, feels different. It might even be showing signs of shadow. My hair is about to start growing back! Just as my darling, sweet friend is preparing to lose hers.

I am visiting her this weekend. It's only a short drive from here and I was able to schedule my appointment early enough in order to get away. Still fascinating and surreal, radiation is becoming routine, and I have no side effects as of yet.

It is difficult to articulate the shock I am feeling, knowing someone so close to me is going through the exact same thing, and all at the same time.

My children are upset, disturbed by the thought of her

suffering. They have seen it firsthand. And I have been hurting, too. But much like facing my own diagnosis, I find myself handling it the same, by sharing with her the cold hard facts of how to deal. There is just no other way.

I know my strength, and I have seen hers as well. But I have also crumbled in fear. It is not fun. Looking back, I understand that it needed to happen, my little three-week episode of thinking the worst. I was barely functioning then, coupled by the actual necessity to do so, treading through daily life with the undue burden of pain and discomfort. The emotional strain is enough to kill you. Forget about the fucking cancer.

I expect to find her in good spirits. She is recovering remarkably well from surgery, light years ahead of my own experience, now nearly a decade ago. Expected to endure a similar course of treatment, her schedule will vary slightly from mine, and everyone responds in different ways. I hope hers comes with much greater ease.

Because the one thought that keeps preying on me is that I should have been enough. Not as some martyr. Believe me, I'd rather complain than keep on suffering. But this cannot continue to happen, especially to those I love. Not to my friends and pray not my family, beloved children of mine. I had hoped to endure so they may not have to.

She has asked for my company to shop for scarves, and I'll share what I no longer need. But mostly I will give to her what I have learned, with all of my love and support.

And I should have been enough.

Love Stacy

The happiest people don't have the best of everything.
They just make the best of everything.

July 17, 2014

Dear Cancer,

Twelve down and twenty-one to go, I have made it past a third of my third phase of treatment.

Keeping busy with friends and excursions, I am feeling signs of life again, both in activity and routine. Giving Dave a break from months of accompaniment, I have started driving myself to radiation, though he sometimes joins me for company. Whether from sheer retirement or the thrill of boredom, I cannot be sure.

I had noticed, when first getting out, that traffic has been particularly bad, often pleading to myself. *Please, please, please, let me get to where I am going.* A rumination on my sickly state. But I am feeling so much better now, both physically and prospectively. Like faithful friends, the two simply go hand in hand.

Still not bothered by side effects, I do feel an occasional tightness in my right side. No more, or less, or different from the general discomfort I've had for years, as a result of my bilateral mastectomy. But don't we all suffer, at some time, from something? I have learned to adjust; to accommodate, to compromise, and to accept what has become a part of my life.

Uncomfortable effects of menopause remain, stifling flashes in hot pursuit. The irony of life frozen in time, yet unable to escape my own heat.

But I am moving forward, catching up, enjoying some peace and getting my rest. And the best is yet to come.

Love Stacy

Life should not be a journey to the grave with the intention of arriving safely in a well-preserved body, but rather to skid in sideways, chocolate in one hand, wine in the other, body thoroughly worn out and screaming "Woo hoo, what a ride!" [9]

July 26, 2014

Dear Cancer,

Fifteen doses in three more weeks and *Hooray!*, I am done. Finished with radiation, the third round of treatment in my second battle with breast cancer. Though my care will never be complete.

I will be fighting this disease every single day for the rest of my life. With each estrogen-blocking pill and every bit

---

9   Uncredited; adapted from the quote by Hunter S. Thomson: "Life should not be
     a journey to the grave with the intention of arriving safely in a pretty and well
     preserved body, but rather to skid in broadside in a cloud of smoke, thoroughly
     used up, totally worn out, and loudly proclaiming 'Wow! What a ride!'"

of my resolve. My chance of recurrence as a BRCA carrier never diminishes, no matter how many years shall pass. It is a difficult truth to embrace.

And so instead, I have let it go. Not a matter of total denial, but the parallel existence of constant survival: I must absolutely liberate myself from fear.

No signs of redness or burning, the area of radiation remains in good condition. I have, it seems, thick skin; earned from experience and toughened by time.

In contrast to my expectations, the days are passing quickly. This summer, so different from years past, has been a respite. For fifteen minutes each day, my treatments have become surprisingly pleasant; a moment of meditation in quiet relief. Enjoying my schedule and its routine, I am occupied. Finally too busy to worry and wonder.

Looking back, I realize I was denied the luxury to do so. Obtaining her driver's license just days after my diagnosis, my daughter was off, and on her own. Keys in one hand, independence in the other. I never had the chance to be concerned, so very consumed in my own conflict. Her freedom, a contrary side effect of my cancer, became an opportunity for growth, however abnormal and unjust.

I have reached that odd place, the forgotten land of what just was. I can hardly remember what this past year was like, and how I got through, now that I am moving so swiftly ahead. We remain active with friends and planning our fall, enjoying time at home and taking pleasure in the ordinary.

And as I am nearing the end, I know once again, it is only the beginning.

Love Stacy

Don't let your struggle become your identity.

July 30, 2014

Dear Cancer,

Hump day and I am hurting a little, my right side sore from the simulation and my skin a bit raw, though no real signs of redness. Looking like a class of kindergartners got hold of some markers and me, the blue crosses and cross sections have been touched up for alignment, with a goofy green line now encircling the six-inch scar below my breast, where the tumor site is targeted for my final boost.

Yesterday, as I sat in the basement waiting for my second simulation, I was reminded this is the same hospital where I've had one, two, three, four, five ... six surgeries for breast cancer; it is the same place where my son was born, eighteen years ago in just two days; my daughter delivered, to everyone's surprise, in the hallway, just twenty minutes after we arrived and without a doctor's supervision; and before that, the very place where I, too, was born. They found my records in the system, as a patient and newborn, when I registered at the age of twenty-six for my own maternity.

It is the place where my mother walked me out of and into this world; the same place where, as a new mother myself, I swaddled my first-born baby boy tightly in two blankets to keep him warm for the ride home, despite the brutal heat of August; where we left with our baby girl just hours after delivery, so swift was her birth; where everyone knew I was undergoing my mastectomy but no one made aware when I went back for a second fight.

As I was leaving, passing by the front doors through which I have come and gone so many times—getting life, giving life, saving life—I was overcome with emotion. The temple of my familiar. I don't know if I love this place or hate it.

At radiation my tech noted that I am in the countdown. Reminded later that day at simulation, they asked how I will celebrate. And again, I just don't know. I am so full of gratitude for my exceptional treatment; for the compassion, concern and care I received from doctors, nurses, and everyone involved. But I have no idea how to commemorate what I hope to leave behind. Nor do I know how I will feel, in only two and a half weeks, other than relieved.

I don't know if fighting breast cancer—again—warrants

celebration, by virtue of being a battle in the first place. It is recurrent and ongoing, and only the end of having to show up. But the beginning of everything else.

And I'm not quite sure how to pick a date to party when every day is cause for celebration.

Love Stacy

Will I become
uncomfortably numb
immobile
black and blue

Will I begin
to move about
and start my life
anew

Will I remain
uncomfortably numb
mere memory of sensation

Or will I forget
this past of mine
and welcome celebration

MARCH 4, 2006

We can't all be princesses. Someone has to clap when I go by.

August 3, 2014

Dear Cancer,

Holy crap, two weeks to go and radiation just hit me like a ton of bricks. Two-hour nap in the day and two-drink maximum at night, and I was rudely awakened this eve, buried under the weight of the world and beneath my own heat, the hot flashes still a regular occurrence, if twenty-four seven is considered routine.

This week showed the signs, radiation rearing its ugly head in the form of fatigue and a big square patch of pink on my chest. My days are not so bad: morning exercise, two meals and my mid-day appointment, followed by afternoon rest and dinner and not much else, the weekends offering a two-day reprieve. But everything feels heavier. I was told this is cumulative and it has finally caught up.

Every day I am X-rayed and zapped, twenty-three treatments

plus three simulations so far. Add in the PET, an MRI, a bone density scan and two views of my spine, and I am soaking in the summer rays. Surely no one really gets it unless they've gotten it themselves.

And in a cruel twist of fortune, my lashes and brows have finally surrendered, giving out just as my hair is coming in. But my spirits are up, even as my body feels weighted down.

I still don't fully understand how treatment works, other than I am full of it. So much radiation residing inside me, I feel like Hiroshima. But just call me hero for short.

Love Stacy

"Take your pleasure seriously."

—CHARLES EAMES

August 5, 2014

Dear Cancer,

Last day of the large field and my blue lines are off! Just eight more rounds to go, in one last final boost. Uplifting, to say the least. This change in treatment should allow for my skin to heal, and though I was feeling low last weekend, I am right back up again. We continue to play and play and play. All I've really done this summer is have fun.

Whether it's in light of the last few months or a settling back into ourselves, we are truly enjoying our time together and especially with friends, and it's hard to believe this will all be over so soon. The sentiment sounds strange, but this has been our life for so many months. All that time, wasted and with purpose, in languish and labor. So much nothingness, yet all of it work.

No guilt in my pleasure, perhaps it's been earned. But I

do not feel deserving so much as appreciative. For life is nothing without joy, nor complete without pain; now on the see and done with the saw. There is so much light at the end of the tunnel.

My son starts this year as a senior in high school, the end of the beginning and the dawn of the end. And so I ponder my story as well: my first diagnosis came nine years ago August, this same month concludes the end of another. Our final chapter before a new book begins.

The finish of radiation marks the start of school, the last bit of summer bittersweet, though my emotions these days are not mixed. I am simply, and truly, happy. Concerned as I was about this treatment, it has been easy, and I must remind myself once again that fear is futile. Worry is always, in all ways, a waste of time.

And though I'll work always so I may survive, in all ways I'll play to stay alive.

Love Stacy

"The trouble is, you think you have time."
—JACK KORNFIELD

August 11, 2014

Dear Cancer,

Around the time of our tenth anniversary, nearly ten years ago, I remember clearly having the impression that we were halfway through. In terms of raising our family, living under the same roof together, half our years were gone. Already. Ethan was about nine years old, Ryan nearly seven. I felt, by all means, a sense of urgency. A recognition that time is fleeting, and the joys of raising young children pass quickly, in the blink of an eye.

Blink. Here we are. My son is eighteen and beginning his last year of high school just days from now.

When I expressed this sentiment to friends, most of us in the same stage of life with children of similar age, they seemed flummoxed. Wondering why I would think such thoughts, or even have time to ponder it, all of us so caught up in the daily grind and ritual of caring for our kids.

Months later, that same year we celebrated our tenth anniversary in January of 2005, I received my first diagnosis.

Perhaps my sense of urgency was unusual. Whether prophetic or practical, who's to say? But I have always felt it, and rightfully so. Hindsight may be twenty-twenty, but my prediction was clear. I don't know if my time is short, but it is most certainly precious, and even without knowing what was to come, I knew that then.

This weekend we had a celebration for Ethan's eighteenth birthday. We delayed the party by a week, waiting for Ryan to return home from her summer travels so we could celebrate collectively, being together ranking higher in priority than celebrating on the actual date. In an ideal world, she would have been here on her brother's birthday, but the world is not ideal. I am forty-four, I have two children still in my care and I have fucking cancer.

Soon I will have to train myself to say I had—not have—cancer, but not until my doc gives me the green light. Permission to say so: I HAD cancer. Twice. Fuck the ideal world.

But back to the party. We gathered my son's closest friends at his favorite place, a fine restaurant we enjoy mostly for special occasions, and during dinner, expressing his concern about the cost, he told me I didn't have to host such a nice event. Of course I didn't have to. I wanted to. This milestone was very important to me, as every birthday, anniversary and significant event has become. Now more than ever.

I explained this to him, that it was my pleasure, and throwing this party was essential to me, especially now. I want him to know how special he is, how very important he is to my life; how lucky I am to have seen him to this age and to have made it to this day.

At forty-four, I am too young to have to wonder how much more time I have with my children; how many more birthdays and milestones we shall pass together. Every celebration is significant, each moment is momentous. My sense of appreciation has been awakened, and my gratitude profound.

In five days, I finish radiation. In five months, we will celebrate our twentieth wedding anniversary. Every celebration is significant. Each moment is momentous. How lucky I am to have made it to this day.

Love Stacy

"Being brave doesn't mean you aren't scared. Being brave means you are scared, really scared, badly scared, and you do the right thing anyway."

—NEIL GAIMAN

August 13, 2014

Dear Cancer,

Number three today. Three out of thirty-three radiation treatments. As in three, two, one.

I can feel it already, the tears starting to well up, waiting to come pouring out, come Friday. All that emotion, every single feeling I've had in the last five months, since that shocking Tuesday afternoon in March when I got the call. I had seen my doctor that morning, a follow-up from the surgery five days before. No pathology results yet, no worries. He had removed a mass at the base of my breast I was sure to be benign. Not cancer. Scar tissue, probably. Something else, maybe. Anything but cancer.

It had never crossed my mind. I knew it was a possibility, but not possibly for me. I'd had a bilateral mastectomy eight and a half years prior. I knew my body. I was in perfect health. I'd done everything right. I had already made the sacrifice.

All those years ago, after my surgery and during the months-long process of reconstruction, I wrote to get through. I wrote and I walked, and I walked and I walked. Ten miles some mornings, just to clear my mind. When the walking wasn't enough, I started to run. I ran and I ran, until I ran the half marathon. Not because I needed to prove anything to anyone, but because it made me feel alive. And I felt good doing it. I was so damn proud of myself for running that race. Still am. Though I'm back to walking, hips don't lie, not needing to prove anything to anyone.

At radiation today I was feeling excited. Two more days and I am done. My treatment will be over. I will ring that bell. I know on Friday I will have done everything I can. Again.

I also know it is no guarantee. I am finished but I am not cured. That is not fear; it's fact. I will be running for the rest of my life.

All I want is to be alive, and to feel good doing it.

Love Stacy

You had the power all along, my dear.[10]

—GLINDA THE GOOD

August 15, 2014

Dear Cancer,

I am DONE. Last radiation treatment and I rang that bell. LOUD. I wanted you all to hear it. I wanted the whole world to hear it. I wanted my heart and my soul and, MY GOD ... HEAR IT. I am done. I am finished. Let this please, please, please be the end.

The day was a bit anticlimactic even though the moment felt significant. I had thought it might be nice to include friends, to have them watch me ring the bell, but it's still summer, many of them traveling or living elsewhere or busy with their lives, and I had a hard time wanting to trouble anyone for such a brief stop in the middle of their day. I'll have to have a party instead.

---

10   Inspired by the quote: "You've always had the power to go back to Kansas," from *The Wizard of Oz*, directed by Victor Fleming (Metro-Goldwyn-Mayer, 1939).

So without fanfare, I was surrounded by the very most important people in my life: David and my two beautiful children, who were almost, just barely, ready to leave on time. Ugh, teenagers … I scheduled my appointment at twelve-thirty just for them.

There were tears to be sure, but as it turns out, I did my crying at home while dressing to leave, overcome by the emotion of this one last time, all those feelings cupped in the hands of conclusion. It was David who cried hard, often emotional when I am steeled, like the two times I received my diagnoses, and particularly this round when they wheeled me in the second time, surgery to make for damn sure all the cancer was out. I love him and know him and understand him more than anyone in this world. Yet I wondered what he was feeling, why those tears were shed. Relief for the end? Joy? Sadness for what I—what we—have been through? Hope for the future? Fear of the unknown?

The reason I was crying this morning actually had little to do with me and everything to do with my family. Because this was never just about me. Of course I want to live a long life. I love my life. I experience so much happiness and joy, from the simplest, everyday pleasures to great and wonderful adventures. Often, and all the time. And I want, selfishly, so much more of that. More of everything, more time for everything. Travel and friendship and fun. Pleasure. Adventure.

But at the end of the day, it was always and only about my family.

I was thinking about my life and how desperately I want more of it. To be here for birthdays and graduations and weddings and milestones, because all of that gives me joy. To be here, especially, for the tough times, too. Heartbreaks and health crises and all the unexpected woes to come.

Because the other side of my selfishness, of my wanting to be here, is not wanting my family to be here without me. All those joys—birthdays, graduations, weddings, milestones; all the fun and friendship and travel; every experience— with my loss, would instead bring sorrow. The bitterness of not being together to enjoy those moments, to support each other in times of struggle. Everything, each milestone, every adventure, any episode of pain, would bring anguish, if I were not here. There would be no comfort in joy, no solace for the ache.

I have suffered. Greatly. But it doesn't matter. It never mattered. It was always just a means to an end. So here I am. Done. Finished. Let this please, please, please be the end.

Love Stacy

Don't take life too seriously.
Nobody gets out alive anyway.

August 18, 2014

Dear Cancer,

Just a few days out from radiation, since I've finished treatment, and I am noticing a lot of the ugly is going away. The scars on my chest from the port, hideous and frustrating to me, are fading. My hair, still indeterminate, is growing back, my lashes and brows returning rapidly.

A few months back, when I was completely bald and my aunt had ignorantly presumed my illness terminal, Dave took a picture of me one afternoon while we were relaxing in bed. He had snapped it on his phone, unbeknownst to me, and sent it to a friend as a joke. The angle was so unbecoming, a shot of the top of my naked head. Lying in repose, I looked unflatteringly—and quite frankly—dead. It was so funny, especially in light of that upsetting message, that we began exchanging emails and texts in reference to my passing. *It happened so fast! This was so unexpected!*

We laughed so hard, we laughed until we cried. It was a good cry. A great release from the stress and disturbance we had recently been experiencing. We were joking about my death, and as a result we had a good time.

It's been almost nine years now since my bilateral mastectomy, since my body has been whole. I am used to the ugly.

But don't get me wrong. I love my body. It is beautiful. Not in the way it once was, and not in the traditional sense. It is now beautiful to me because of experience, and for being loved. Instead of the glory of youth, its beauty comes from the good fortune of age. Every day I get older, I get luckier, too.

I was a bit more tired this past weekend, exhausted from the emotion of the end, and partly some weariness to be expected. The effects of radiation are cumulative and will stay with me for about four more weeks, I am told. But today is my first "free" day.

Free from treatment. Free from cancer. Free from fear.

I am alive. I am ALIVE. I AM ALIVE!

Love Stacy

Always tight and quite upright
That is my new condition
But consider it reversely
And I'll take the better option

For always right and quite uptight
Is rather unbecoming
And although this chest is not my own
The figure I am loving!

MAY 22, 2006

Love more, worry less.

August 25, 2014

Dear Cancer,

My very best friend in high school had an older brother who was cute, smart and popular, a star athlete at our school. She and I came from different neighborhoods and religious backgrounds, but we adored each other. We had other things in common: her parents divorced, mine were perpetually divorcing; we were given, coincidentally, the same car upon our sixteenth birthdays; we met in middle school but became close during high school where we had both transferred as magnet students.

I had always idealized her family dynamic: one boy, one girl. Older brother, younger sister. Though I never fully envisaged my future of marriage and family, I remember wanting a boy and a girl, in that idyllic teenage dream sort of way. And then I grew up and it came true.

I never imagined my happily married life, mostly because I never witnessed one. It just happened, and I am both lucky and grateful for it. Admittedly, I presumed cancer was in my future because of my strong family history, but not at thirty-five. And certainly not twice.

There are certain things we imagine that manifest; dreams that are realized either by hard work, or chance, or both. Other realizations we never could have envisioned that transpire, forming our lives. But many of these aspirations are, ultimately, beyond our control. Timing, luck, circumstance. All of these factors are what predict our futures, even more than our hopes and dreams, teenage or otherwise.

For all my predictions, I have always believed I would live a long life. It's just something I had generally sensed. And I won't say that has changed. But I have.

Cancer has changed me. It didn't the first time, but it has now. I can't help but question what my future holds, and not in the normal way of wonder.

It feels like I no longer have my feet planted firmly on the ground. Instead I live in an ocean, constantly having to keep my head above water, lest I drown in fear. Sometimes I float easily, without worry. Other times I am exhausted by the unknown. The sea is vast, and I am always surrounded.

Tomorrow I meet with the oncologist, my first follow-up since chemotherapy and radiation. I don't know what, exactly, to expect. I'm sure we will discuss my protocol, the type and frequency of testing. I know David is hoping for an all-clear, though he knows there is really no way to know for sure. I just want to clear my mind.

My doctor will probably begin my course of endocrine therapy, a maintenance drug which is the most critical part of prevention. Ten more years of treatment and side effects, some unpleasant, others detrimental. But she hopes it is lifesaving, and I am hoping for the best.

Over the years, distance has grown between my friend and me, though we are still in touch. Our lives parted in various directions; some by choice, others by chance. I don't know if our dreams were different but our hopes are all the same: to live long and healthy lives. And I know she wishes me the best.

Love Stacy

"Be so good they can't ignore you."

—STEVE MARTIN

August 29, 2014

Dear Cancer,

Every time I get up in the middle of the night, I break out in a hot flash. I'm not sure why. They are triggered for sure, and the movement must spark their interest. Last night, after going to the bathroom for the nth time, I returned to bed, trying to cool off by flipping my pillow. Flipping and flopping, twisting and turning, unable to find the cool side. I was simply too hot.

When Ryan was born and Ethan was only nineteen months old, I remember lying in bed nursing her while Ethan sat on the floor eating a yogurt. I was no longer hands free, and instead of depending on me for help he figured it out, sitting at the coffee table in my bedroom, holding a spoon and feeding himself. It was a small task but a moment monumental, and one I will never forget. My sweet little boy, at only one and a half, was spreading his wings. Now he's applying for college.

Our first home was a townhouse in a growing arts district. The master bedroom was so large that it became over the years an all-purpose room, first with a sitting area used as a living spot, then crowded with toys and the general detritus of our young family. It was, for all intents and purposes, my children's game room, with a tool center for Ethan and mini kitchen nearby for the both of them.

We had a small yard in front, walking distance to art galleries and Whole Foods, before Whole Foods exploded into the ether of culture, and walking distance being relative, me being the only mother as if in New York who treated this town as urban. Baby joggers were also new back in the day of my children's youth, and so I had two. The first one for Ethan, then a double for my two under two, and I used those strollers for everything, including a grocery cart. I would walk to the store with both kids in tow, stuffing my groceries in the back pockets until checkout. A hippie at Whole Foods before hipsters were cool. It was a sweet time, long before the use of cell phones, and I loved being—literally—hands free.

At my recent follow-up, the doctor said I am cancer-free, and she seemed to have no concern for my future. The aromatase inhibitor—estrogen blocker for short—can cause joint pain, but four doses in and so far so good. Three thousand six hundred and forty-six pills to go. She said yoga and stretching will help, should I develop discomfort over time, but I'm not so worried anymore. After all, I seem to have beaten radiation rather than it beating me; still exercising every day, and with no lingering fatigue. I am grateful for the little things.

The underbelly of my right breast is still burned, so I apply aloe each night as directed, and one recent evening, after taking a quick walk and subsequent shower before dinner, I came downstairs to prepare our meal with my shirt only half on, allowing the ointment to dry. It was neither appropriate nor offensive, my family accepting of my antics when it comes to my needs. But my daughter noticed something unusual. "I didn't know mom has abs." *Well, we all have abs, honey.* I guess mine showed more definition than expected, my stomach the final frontier of a body intact. Nothing else looks the same.

Her funny remark made me feel good, and I was flattered.

Maybe I am a cool mom. Hot. Like the flip side of the pillow.

Love Stacy

"Be patient and tough; someday this pain will be useful to you."

—OVID

September 3, 2014

Dear Cancer,

For several weeks now, the road outside our street has been under construction. We live on a cul-de-sac and it is the only access in and out of our quiet corner. We drive in circles around the neighborhood to get on and off our street, and the congestion is so bad we are often stuck, waiting minutes on end while trucks maneuver in order for us to enter or exit. My car is covered in mud, our driveway lined and garage thickly layered with dust.

The other day, as I approached the intersection, I saw before me a massive pile of dirt with a sign propped in front: One Way. As if we had a choice. One side of the access road has been dug into a deep culvert, the other lane is crumbling away.

I had to stop and take pause. There before my eyes was a giant metaphor of my life. An enormous pile of shit in front of me and only one way to get through.

It will be months before the construction is complete.

Today marks the nineteenth anniversary of Angela's death, David's sister and my beloved friend who died unexpectedly and suddenly at the age of twenty-six. In the wake of her loss, we became who we are.

It is the same date I received my first diagnosis, precisely ten years after her death, and nine years ago this week. I awoke today feeling not myself, my body and joints not unhappy, but less so. If not the effects of medication, then it is my history accumulating.

I've been patient with the construction, dealing with the delays, unconcerned by the mess, and appreciative of the men plowing away in the difficult heat. Their efforts will improve our city, and I am grateful for their hard work.

I have learned through the years to accept what has been lost, to be patient with the process, to avoid the ditches and drive right on through, passing all those piles of dirt. And I am so very grateful.

It is the one and only way.

Love Stacy

We are living our adventure.

September 16, 2014

Dear Cancer,

I used to be a screamer.

Take a moment, get your mind out of the gutter, and allow me to rephrase. I used to raise my voice, yell at my kids. Not a lot, but more than I would like to admit, and certainly more than I would have liked to do. And then one day, many years ago, I stopped. I don't know if they got easier to parent or I got better at parenting, but my rage began to dissipate, to seep away with time.

I still get firm in tone, and I have always been loud, a flaw of which I am well aware and cannot seem to change. But there is a difference between making yourself heard and losing your shit, and it is not a fine line. It's a giant gap.

The truth is I was raised to yell. I raised hell as a kid. Not in a rebellious way, but because my mother and I fought, tooth and nail, nearly every single day. Not in starts and fits—there was always a fit. She was full of fury, both a flaw in character and consequence of her frustrated marriage to my dad. But ours was the most complicated of relationships. We simply never saw eye to eye.

To her credit, she stopped yelling one day, too, but it was long after I was gone, out of the house and away from the chaos of my parents' life, and probably the result of many sessions in therapy. I have never sought that kind of help, nor do I hold her responsible for my own behavior. That is the beauty of becoming an adult: we are each accountable for our actions, for the person we choose to be.

It is amazing how very deeply we are affected by our parents, no matter how many years separate us from our upbringing, though my experience does not fill me with resentment, or even sadness for that matter. Instead it brings to me awareness, a keen reminder every day of who I am as a mother and wife, and how I parent and love. It is, in the labyrinth that is life, the very gift I was given, my lesson learned, from the parents who raised me—with love—in an environment so vastly filled with pain.

This evening I was awakened abruptly, David stirring me from a dream. I was yelling in my sleep, trapped in a nightmare I could not escape, until he brought me out, shaking me back into consciousness. I have always been plagued by dreams, extremely vivid in-living-color experiences, some which I have been able to recall, with clarity, for many, many years. Intense and complex stories I could convert into fantasy or film, if only I had the capacity to do so.

Many of my dreams, if not most, are manifestations of my fears. Visually affected, I am careful not to watch horror or violence, but scenes from the news, memories past, residual tidbits from the everyday all seem to visit me at night. And now I have the nightmare of my reality.

This past weekend we took a trip, five couples getting away for fun, and fun was had by all. We also gathered to celebrate our friend's birthday, the one who is, too, battling breast cancer. It was not a particular milestone though each year is important. And we got to talking about how we will celebrate, together, our fiftieth birthdays.

We share, all of us, a great mutual friendship; each of us friends with the other, each spouse in love with their other. Friends we count as family, the folks we want to grow old with. I am, not always but often, the youngest among my peers, as is the case with this group. And here is my dirty little secret.

Every time, every single time anyone mentions fifty, no matter who, when, where or what, no matter the happy or mad circumstance, all I can think is this: *Will I make it? Will I make it to fifty?* That is more than five years from now. Six to be precise, and don't get me started with statistics. I shouldn't even say it, but I think it. All the time. Fifty. It seems right around the corner. For many of us, it is. But it's an eternity for me.

That is the demon of this disease. My days have, for the most part, returned to normal. I have some aches and pains, but I try not to wear them on my sleeve. I feel pretty good, I look pretty good, but here at the strip center, behind the attractive façade, is a little shop of horrors. No one can see what's under my shirt, what's hiding inside my mind. How difficult it is to live with the devil.

In the course of all the fun from our recent vacation, I am in the midst of a rough week. Awaiting incomplete results from a PET scan last week, and living day to day with the general unknown of this awful disease, I have four follow-up appointments this week and I am keeping it all together. But that which goes unseen in the light reveals itself by dark. And so tonight I woke up screaming.

It was so wonderful to get away this weekend; to have some fun and keep on living. I realized last week that what I need most right now is distance. Distance from this fucking disease, time away from my reality. A goddamn break from the misery of it all. Because time is the answer. It is the only thing to separate me from my disease. The only factor that will get me to fifty.

In the meantime, we are carping the fuck diem.

Fuck you cancer. You fucking fuck.

Love Stacy

I would like to apologize to anyone I have not offended. Please be patient. I will get to you shortly.

September 18, 2014

Dear Cancer,

Last night the truth came out. We were sitting at dinner, as we do together every night, almost without exception, and my son said I use the F-word too much. He was, to our mutual understanding, referring to my Facebook posts. My husband agreed, "It's a bit much."

"Yeah, Mom," echoed my daughter.

I conceded.

And then I asked her if she reads my posts, because I really wasn't sure. David and my son acknowledge them in the traditional way, but my girl ... not so far as I could tell. She said if she likes a post, it would show up on her feed and notify her friends. All twelve hundred and thirty-six of them.

I know I have put my life—and therefore hers—on display, for all the world to see. She isn't fooling anyone, and she knows it.

I don't talk the way I write, at least not often, and rarely around my kids. I am venting and they get it. This is my way out. And I make no apologies.

But I am sorry for their pain.

Before bed my son came to my room, as he always does, to kiss me and say goodnight, and he substantiated his earlier complaint. He said he understands why I choose that word. He knows I use it for emphasis, which is exactly why it upsets him so much.

It hurts him to see my sorrow, to feel my struggle, to know my truth.

Only recently have I begun to break through my shell of the past six months. To re-emerge slowly into the world, to see through the bubble of hell I've been living in. To consider what these last miserable months have been like for David, and for my beautiful kids.

Not in response to my son's sensitive words, but because I finally realized how selfish I have been in my experience. Lost in my life to my very own suffering, unable to consider anyone else, not even the needs of those most in need. The thought of my children losing their mother, my husband bereaving his wife.

I cannot imagine what it's like for a child, to know what goes on inside of their minds.

I've been trying lately to put myself in David's shoes, to question how he must be feeling, and coping with all of this mess. His fear of losing me, his frustration with the process. Is he mad at my body for causing me harm? Angry at how this has altered our life? Does he resent me for my illness, or my illness for me?

My daughter recently grumbled that we had not had a real dinner in days. By that she meant we did not sit down as a family for several nights last week, forgetting that she was dismissed for a rare evening practice, Dave at a meeting and absent another, even though meals were prepared. Two nights in a row without us together and she was distressed.

We are used to routine, accustomed to each other. And the earth has been shattered under their feet.

I wondered if I could replace all the F-bombs with something benign. A cure for the cancer of my words. If I could edit my experience, and make the world a safer place.

Dear Cancer, you stupid.

Stupid, stupid you.

Love Stacy

> *"Sometimes you just need to take a nap and get over it."*
>
> —MAURA STUARD, AGE 8

September 24, 2014

Dear Cancer,

Nightmare number five. Tonight is the fifth time in the last two weeks I have been awakened. Sobbing, screaming, shaking, sweating. My brain is mush, my body a ball of nerves. I am altogether coming apart.

The PET scan results are in; neither good nor definitively bad. An MRI ordered next week to clarify metastasis once and for all. As my oncologist brazenly stated, "to put the beast to rest."

I am living with a monster.

If the cancer were in my spine indeed, I would feel it, I am told. But I am not in pain.

I could—perhaps I should—be taking medication to get some rest, to ease the anxiety, but I'm afraid if I start, I will never be able to stop. Dependent on my desire to escape, and I have never, ever felt this way before. Dread like in the beginning except this is supposed to be the end.

The other four letter F-word. And one I will not say.

But I can feel it in my bones.

Love Stacy

"Sometimes your only available transportation is a leap of faith."

—MARGARET SHEPARD

September 30, 2014

Dear Cancer,

MRI today and it wasn't so bad, the cacophonous barrage a pleasant distraction from the usual noise inside my head.

Gently put, these last three weeks have been trying. Testing, waiting, wonder. Repeat. A vicious cycle of torment. We didn't talk about the tension, but it was sharp like a knife.

First the wait and further the worry.
My heart and head were all a flurry.
Then came the call. On my knees, will I fall?
There is no cancer upon your spine
You are going to be, my dear, just fine.

Trauma, trauma, of the mind.

At long last, we can all take a deep breath. Put our weapons down.

Outside of my street, the familiar mess of construction has become ever more complicated and frustrating. And then today, day of all days, a welcome coincidence as they poured concrete and re-paved the road. A stronger foundation, a new beginning.

Finally, another way out.

I can start to put one foot in front of the other.

To get back on the road again. And drive.

Love Stacy

"Do the best you can until you know better. Then when you know better, do better."

—MAYA ANGELOU

October 2, 2014

Dear Cancer,

This afternoon I was running a quick errand, picking up clothes from the dry cleaners about a mile or so from my house, when on the sidewalk I spotted the teeny tiniest little two-wheeler, with hot pink handles and tassels to boot, and on it the cutest little girl just peddling away. This bicycle was so small, I took a moment to consider the absence of training wheels. Impressive. Farther ahead was the parent, leaving just enough space to foster independence, allowing the child to follow behind. It was the sweetest thing I'd ever seen.

As I pulled closer to the stop sign, I realized the dad was my neighbor—and one of my dearest friends. Earlier this year, his wife had taken off work to sit through a day of chemo with me.

I slowed down to say hello, not yet coming to a stop, and all of a sudden, *HONK!!*

A long, loud, get-out-of-my-way siren. And then the drive-by. A raging, running-through-the-stop-sign pull-around and pass. This asshole of a woman was in such a rush, she didn't care that she had frightened a child, startled us adults, raced through an intersection and broken the law.

So I followed her. She happened to turn the corner and pull right into a bank, just as I had assumed she might, and there was an open lane next to her in the drive through. She was a classy looking lady, in a lovely luxury car, with a beautiful, dainty diamond cross around her neck. And she had no excuse.

I got out of my car and gave her a piece of my mind. It was not a shining moment for me, but if I made her feel bad, then I did my good deed for the day.

I do not understand why people are so impatient. In a hurry sometimes, I understand. But angry and mean and disrespectful and dangerous? I just don't get it. What a fucking bitch.

And I'm the one who's had cancer. Twice. Imagine being the patient.

Life is not fair, but why make it miserable? Pause. Calm down. Appreciate the sweet and small things, like beautiful children on little pink bikes. The great and the grand, like good health and life.

Make the world a better place. A peaceful place. Slow down. Be kind.

Go big or go home.

Love Stacy

Being fabulous is the best revenge.

October 13, 2014

Dear Cancer,

One week past my last procedure, a minor surgery to revise the scar from my port, still itching, throbbing and hurting all these months since it was removed, and I am finally starting to get some space. Not yet the distance I need, but a break.

It's like the bad boyfriend, the one you know isn't good for you but you just can't seem to break it off, end it, get him out of your life. And then he goes away for a little while. Say, on business or to see his family ... or to screw some other girl.

And you realize how refreshing his absence really is—how good it feels to feel like yourself again.

Before the end of this year, I have two more follow-ups, with the radiation oncologist and my main squeeze medical oncologist, plus a repeat MRI and PET scan to make sure everything remains stable. Another week of anticipation and stress, and then it's over. The end of this year. The final break up.

Dear Cancer,

We are never, ever, ever getting back together.

Like, ever.

Love Stacy

"Look closely at the present you are constructing: it should look like the future you are dreaming."

—ALICE WALKER

October 23, 2014

Dear Cancer,

This past weekend, as part of breast cancer awareness month, our school held a ceremony before the high school football game to recognize survivors. For such a small community, there were a disproportionate number of us.

We were called out onto the field and presented with pink roses. We stood together for the national anthem and a few pictures were taken. It was lovely and brief, and instead of looking forward to it, I was stressed out while getting ready.

I am a survivor loud and clear, but I do not wear my status on my sleeve. No pink ribbons, no flamingos in my yard. Not a cheerleader for the cause, just a voice for the experience.

I was grateful for the honor. This has been a difficult year and my battle is most recent. But as I was rushing to get dressed, I realized my hope is to be remembered for who I am and what I have done, not for what has happened to me.

This morning while my daughter was getting ready for school, she yelled down the hall, slight panic in her voice, to ask if there were any clean uniform skirts. I have been so busy, with all good things, that laundry was washed but not folded. Life is getting back to normal.

Yet there is so much collateral damage.

A week after my scar revision the area responded with great irritation, and I suffered from uncontrollable itching for a week. My right breast, growing tighter from radiation, is now causing pain under my arm. Encapsulation. The scarring has begun.

My hair down there and everywhere, pissed from being poisoned, has come back with a vengeance. I even grew a beard. The fuzz was so unruly, Dave had to trim my neck and when I thanked him, he said, "You're welcome, sir."

It was so funny, I can't fault him for the insult. His comic relief is my salve. This is hard for him, too.

It wasn't until a few days after the football game that I remembered. Last Saturday was October 18th, the anniversary of my bilateral mastectomy. It's been nine years. I am usually reminded on this date of the great turning point in my life, even though my diagnosis came several months prior to surgery.

The day passed quietly. Forgotten. A whisper of my past.

Instead of looking back, I am moving ahead, and starting over once again.

Love Stacy

"What we see depends mainly on what we look for."

—JOHN LUBBOCK

November 19, 2014

Dear Cancer,

Two. Only two hot flashes in the last twenty-four hours and that is a record low. Just like the weather, perhaps its due. This latest flash late night awakened me like thunder.

Still on the roller coaster, most days are fun, but some a bit rough. A wave of fear that feels like nausea washes over me on occasion. The unexpected drop or turn, it simply cannot be avoided once you are strapped in and on the ride. But this is no amusement, take my word.

Both PET and MRI are confirmed for December. I was hoping just one would do the work but both tests are needed, to revisit a variety of matters. My back for a third look, plus my liver and lung, the latest to light up on that second exam. The follow-up now forcing me to be followed. Precaution only is what I believe. But it is unnerving in every way.

There sits on the counter in every room of my doctor's clinic a standing book of diagrams, like a giant Rolodex, each page describing every category of cancer and its corresponding stages. Hers always rests on one of the four belonging to breast, but all the tabs are there. I know so much more about this disease than I ever thought I would learn, yet I still don't seem to understand enough.

I am feeling mostly good these days, stronger and more energetic with a few aches and pains I could live without, except that I can't. Probably an effect from the maintenance drug though I am faring better than expected.

Every time something new presents I worry it is here for good, concerned for my long-term health and quality of life. A running muse on my mind. Three weeks of pain and I thought it was permanent, that pesky tightness under my arm. But I worked and worked on working it out, and then one day it disappeared. Mysteriously here and magically gone. Cancer, forever playing its tricks.

And so it goes. My days are here and then they are gone.

Normal and noisy, happy and hopeful. I am running along, reality right behind.

I just keep on keeping on. Catch me if you can.

Love Stacy

I will hold myself to a standard of grace, not perfection.

November 28, 2014

Dear Cancer,

This week I completed the first three months of my mainte-nance drug. One-fortieth of my treatment. Nine years and nine months to go. The medication I'm on is restricted to post-menopausal women, an endocrine therapy designed to block the production of estrogen. Good to the very last drop. Menopause, not on coffee but on crack. My skin is thinning, my joints come wither. I am literally drying up.

I have swallowed hundreds upon hundreds of pills, some with side effects so severe, saboteurs to my health, that I am required to take other drugs to counteract. Remember the steroids to prep for poison, anti-nausea to navigate chemo? Probiotics for my belly, softeners for my stool? Antihistamines to block the pain from Neulasta, used to whip my marrow into making white blood cells. Narcotics to numb. Supplements to save. Now a booster for my bones.

Pro-this, anti-that. A merry-go-round of misery. And finally I have jumped off. Dizzy, but done.

I recently got my very first haircut, for the second time in my life. It's coming in fast and fairly cute, a little bit curly without a streak of grey. Not even chemo could age my color, yet young enough to have cancer twice.

The comments are flowing about my hair, but I cannot stand the critiques. It is a work in progress, but so am I. My hair has changed, and so have I. But I am here. I'm alive. Isn't that all anyone should care about?

To stop and think, for just a moment, about what I have endured? To consider, with compassion, that this is all beyond my control? The cancer, the curls. Whether or not I am cured.

Pay me a compliment or keep it to yourself.

And so the mentions made me count. I have been to a hospital or clinic more than ninety times this year. Scores and scores of separate trips. Endless emails, continuous calls. Appointments to schedule, prescriptions to pick up. Parking and paying, planning and praying. A total consumption of care.

Someone asked me today what I do for a living and I wanted to say: *I live.*

I LIVE. That is what I do. *I live for a living.* That has become my work. Every day I live. Every day I survive. Every day I stay alive.

I live and I love and I love my life.

I am finding my days closer to normal, further and farther away from disease. A little more peace, one day at a time. I am not thankful today because it's Thanksgiving. I am thankful because I'm alive. Grateful for every day of my life, and not in some grand cliché. I am surviving with hope, happy with life, and trying to live with grace.

Love Stacy

*"the most wasted of all
days is one without laughter."*

—E.E. CUMMINGS

December 14, 2014

Dear Cancer,

Hanukkah is coming and in that all-American way I will decorate my home. Not with tinsel and lights but with hanging homemade stars, constructed together with my kids when they were toddlers. A box of colored popsicle sticks, some glue and string on a fall afternoon, and there we were, creating tokens of childhood.

All stored away in one tidy container, today I will unload our box of decorations: ceramics and artwork from their pre-school years, a wrinkled banner and not much else. I have neither added to nor edited our collection in fifteen years, but every holiday it grows a bit sweeter, the farther we are from those innocent days. No cancer, just crafts.

The holiday starts in only two days and I have nothing, not one thing, to wrap for my children. Our gifts are understood this year. I felt guilty this morning, not having any presents to prepare, reminiscing on the days when each night held surprise, both big and small. But I warned my kids and was forgiven. My children have everything they need.

I have not yet arrived at a place of peace, troubled these past few days. My scans are scheduled for later this week. I wish I could say that I live with ease, but that is simply not the truth. I have pesky bad dreams and worrisome thoughts, besotted with concern. My results will come at the end of this year, and I am ready to usher it out.

One of the drawings I've saved in our box has on it a tree with no limbs. No leaves, no green, just a wide, brown trunk, and hysterically phallic it is. I'm not sure which one of my kids drew this masterpiece. No name was written on the back. We have tried for years to figure it out but no one remembers who made the mistake. It's the funniest sketch I've ever seen.

Across the top of the page reads one lonely word, for which celebration we cannot be sure. "Happy," it says. "Happy." That's all. Not Happy Hanukkah, nor Happy New Year. Just … happy. Every year I pull out this picture and tape it to the wall. Every year we laugh again, perplexed, confused and tickled with joy. I should frame it one of these days.

It shall be our family crest. A motto of sorts. A coat of arms. My shield.

A lesson and a gift.

Not the kind to be ribboned or wrapped, but received and cherished and kept.

Happy. I will be happy. It doesn't matter for what.

Love Stacy

"Wherever you are, be all there."

—JIM ELLIOTT

December 19, 2014

Dear Cancer,

Today I feel grateful. I feel a lot of other things, too. But mostly I am grateful. Not for having cancer, or fighting cancer, or beating cancer. Not for me, or my luck, or my life. But for all the people who have loved me, supported me, cared for me, and thought of me throughout this year.

For everyone who listened to me cry, and made me laugh. For everyone who called, texted, emailed, wrote. Liked.

For the ones who always knew what to say, and for those who didn't but tried anyway.

The greatest gift anyone can give is kindness. It is also the easiest. And free. It goes such a long way that it has brought me here. All the way to this day.

And for that, I say thank you.

Love Stacy

Every thought has meaning
Every prayer a gentle hug
Your calls, good luck and wishes
Each one, a sign of love

JANUARY 18, 2007

"It's a funny thing about life; if you refuse to accept anything but the best, you very often get it."

—W. SOMERSET MAUGHAM

December 30, 2014

Dear Cancer,

The Dom is in the fridge.

I love champagne. I have always loved champagne. Not because I'm supposed to, or because it's fancy, or because of tradition. I just love it.

Years ago, before cancer, before anything, Dave always said he was going to serve champagne at his funeral. Not that he could actually tend the bar, if it was his funeral. But he's going to make sure it's there. So we will celebrate his life. He wants everyone to have fun.

I'm not planning my funeral. Not yet. All my scans were clear.

So relieved, I cried.

It's been a long and stressful six weeks. I was doing great, moving on, feeling my life getting back to normal. But once the scheduling began ... the dozens and dozens of emails, back and forth to clarify which tests were needed, and when, and whether or not I could have them on the same day; and once that was cleared, to determine whether I could have only one IV administered for both tests, instead of two separate IVs because that was causing anxiety; and then to see if I could keep the IV in my arm from the morning appointment and travel with it to the afternoon exam, because the tests were administered in different locations.

So, yeah, November was stressful. And then anticipating the scans in December was upsetting. And then awaiting results was, well, somewhat shy of torture. It's just that way.

I was stressed, on high alert. Anxious. And then, knowing that being stressed wasn't good for me, I was upset for being stressed in the first place.

Wasn't it me who said worry is a waste of time?

I wished I could help it, but I couldn't wish it away.

Every time my back hurt or ached, every time I imagined

that it hurt or ached, I worried. *Is this normal? Is it real? Is the pain psychosomatic?* Which in my house means crazy.

Dave has promised to die in the winter when it's cool, not summer when it's too hot to stand outside. No sweating at his ceremony. He wants a Tempur-Pedic mattress to lie upon and insists on being buried with his body tilted upward, since our gravesite is on a hill and he's afraid of drowning. Even when he's dead. But who's calling who crazy?

I have started to understand in these last few months, when I should have been on the mend but was suffering instead, that post-traumatic stress is real. Maybe not PTSD, but post-cancer diagnosis disorder. Normal concerns feel heightened, awareness becomes anxiety.

Because the cancer was there and I didn't know it, and knowing I can't know doesn't mean it isn't there.

But it's over now. Everything is fine. I am done with scans. No more testing. Goodnight, bad dreams. Goodbye, irrational thoughts.

Hello, life.

On any given day, we have a dozen bottles of champagne

stocked in our house. But the Dom Perignon is special. We save it for exceptional occasions. Important events. Birthdays. Anniversaries. New Year's Eve.

Celebrations.

A new year. A new life.

Cheers!

Love Stacy

Be your own kind of beautiful.

January 23, 2015

Dear Cancer,

Today I felt the shift.

Finally, I finally let go. If only for a moment, I was able to let go.

Let go of the struggle.

The fear is fading, but the struggle is always there. Here, with me. Pain. Frustration. Discomfort. Concern.

Disappointment.

My life has changed, my body is altered. And I've been there before. Done that. But now I am changing. Me, the woman I am. The maintenance drug I'm on, the tiny little tablet that is supposed to save me, is also killing me. The love thief, stealing beauty from my life.

A part of me is missing and it's not the missing parts.

My hair, on the other hand, is nothing if not gone astray. It is growing so fast, so wildly unruly, that I must not only learn to embrace it, but to tame it, too.

The other day, after my workout and with no other plans for the afternoon, I decided to try out a new do. I showered, put on pajamas, and with a handful of styling cream, rearranged my hair. A wait and see. And then my son came home.

"Oh my god, what is that?!?" he cried. "You look like a boxer!"

I had slicked back my locks and let it dry, but it puffed up anyway. Whether he meant the dog or a fighter, I'm not to be sure, but we laughed and we laughed. And we laughed some more.

So life goes on. The world keeps spinning, the cycle of life precariously hanging on. Since the start of this year, we've celebrated our twentieth wedding anniversary and we've buried a grandmother. We have laughed and remembered, commemorated and cried. The end of my treatment, the beginning of a new year. A restart of my life, the end of another.

A beginning and an end. An end and a beginning.

Two years ago I participated in a yoga challenge called *Forty Days to Personal Revolution*.[11] It is an opportunity to practice daily yoga and meditation; to go deep, into self-awareness, and self-care. To find your true self. To transform. It may sound hokey, or indulgent. But I have been practicing yoga for nearly seventeen years and it has saved my life. Twice. And every single day.

This year I signed up again. To set myself free.

Free from fear. Free from pain. Free from frustration, discomfort, concern. Disappointment.

Hair envy.

And it's working. Day thirteen and I am feeling it. I am feeling alive, and well, and transformed.

Lucky number thirteen. I was married on the thirteenth. Friday, January 13th, twenty years ago this month. We remembered and celebrated. We commemorated and cried.

I am going to find myself. Again.

Love Stacy

---

11   Baptiste, Baron. *40 Days to Personal Revolution*. Simon & Schuster: New York, 2004.

A true love story never ends.

March 3, 2015

Dear Cancer,

Today is the last day of the first year since my second diagnosis of cancer.

One year ago today I was last at peace. I had cancer in my body, but had no idea. No suspicion, no expectation. I was blissfully ignorant, and therefore free.

I've spent the last three days at a spa with a friend. We share the same birthday and had been planning to celebrate this way, now on an eight-month delay. These were the days we could both get away, and it is not lost on me as the perfect way to conclude my most difficult year. The setting is serene, we are cherished in friendship. I am at peace.

Life begins … now. I will always be in recovery. Always healing. But life begins now. Tomorrow is the beginning of year two. It is an anniversary, no doubt. My life will forever be measured from this moment forward.

This year closes no less emotionally than its treacherous start. Two weeks ago, we unexpectedly lost our beloved dog Lucky. He was the great love of my life and left a hole in my heart the size of a dachshund. Twenty-four hours after saying goodbye, my son Ethan called with his own big news. He was admitted to his first choice of college, the only university he has ever wanted to attend, and it was no small achievement. From one sweet boy to another, sobs of grief to tears of joy, all in a matter of moments. This is the pendulum of my life.

When I was first diagnosed the second time around, several thoughts kept spinning on the turntable of my mind. A broken record of fear. I worried that my dogs would see the death of me and not the other way around. That our grandmothers, both in their late nineties, would outlive me. That my parents, together for twenty-seven miserable years, would have a longer marriage than my happy one. Irrational perhaps, but cancer makes you crazy. Injustices made possible by my anxious mind.

But order has been restored. My dog is dead. Our grandmother is gone. This year we crossed a marriage milestone.

I am healing. And I have found peace. Somehow, in the chaos of life, among the grief and unfairness of it all, I am grounded again. And happy.

I loved a dog and raised a boy. Our grandmother preceded me and we celebrate her life.

I am healing. I have found peace. Order has been restored.

Love Stacy

"Hardship often prepares an ordinary person for an extraordinary destiny."

—CHRISTOPER MARKUS

March 15, 2015

Dear Cancer,

A year ago yesterday, I missed my daughter's sweet sixteen birthday party.

A year ago yesterday, I was under the knife for six hours.

A year ago yesterday, I did not know if I had a fighting chance against this disease.

Yesterday, I made it to our best friend's birthday party.

Yesterday, I was in a car for six hours driving to and from his house.

Yesterday, I didn't even think about a year ago yesterday.

I am so less consumed with this disease. Relieved to know the further the distance, the faster it is growing.

It wasn't until I opened Facebook that I remembered to think about a year ago yesterday. I received a notification that my page got a new Like.

Nine hundred and seventy-eight to date. I don't care. And I'm not counting.

It's not the numbers I have received. It's the love. You have helped me heal.

I am going to do something with all of this. I'm not sure how and I don't know when. But I am.

So help me break a thousand.

If you haven't liked my page yet, please, Like it. I will love you for it back.

Love Stacy

"You are the poem I never knew how to write and this life is the story I have always wanted to tell."

—TYLER KNOTT GREGSON

April 15, 2015

Dear Cancer,

For the first time in my life I spent two and a half hours at Whole Foods and didn't spend a dime. Today I went to write. To be alone, to think in peace, in a perfect, quiet place. Outdoor seating, indoor air conditioning, food, water and restrooms. Check.

I am a sucker for Whole Foods. I love it. Overpriced produce, grains in bulk, chocolate and cheeses, beer and bread. Grass fed beef and fresh caught fish. Organic almost everything. I once bought a jar of marinara that cost only $6.00. The year was 1989.

I don't do all of my shopping there. In fact, I don't do any grocery shopping anymore. Dave took over that responsibility last year and I never took it back. But I have been going to Whole Foods since the very first store opened on Lamar Boulevard in Austin, Texas, when I was a student at UT. My son begins there this fall.

I used to stop in Whole Foods when we were building our first house and I needed a place to go for a break. It has always been home base. Now I'm using it to get away, to think and remember and write. I have a story to tell.

The shift I felt months ago and the place where I landed feels firm. I am no longer plagued with fear. I think of you often, how every good thought might have killed every bad cell, and I thank you for all of the love.

So please bear with me. I do not want to speak too soon, or out of turn, or not at all. Stick around. This is going to be good.

Love Stacy

"You have power over your mind—not outside events. Realize this, and you will find strength."

—MARCUS AURELIUS

May 21, 2015

Dear Cancer,

This week we lost the last of our grandmothers, my sweet Grammy Gert. She was ninety-seven years and ten months old, and yes, those ten months count. Because every day counts.

My grandmother was an exceptional woman, loving and kind, funny and fashion-forward. She raised four daughters and was the hippest of them all. For twenty-seven years, Grammy lived independently and alone, since the passing of my Grandpa David, her beloved husband of fifty-two years. She worked and drove until just last year and volunteered in the hospital regularly, including the Friday before she passed. She made the best damn gumbo on either side of the Mississippi and she lived a full and vibrant, healthy life until the moment of her death. At her funeral someone remarked that she once said she'd had pneumonia when she was four years old and was never sick another day in her life. On Sunday morning she suddenly died while peacefully in bed.

One of my cousins said that our grandmother divorced herself from negativity and loved her family in all its manifestations, and I knew this as the beautiful truth. She was joyful and happy and loved us all, and I felt her love, no matter what. As we were leaving the funeral another one of my cousins said she believed our Grammy lived such a healthy, long life because she was always a positive person. It was also the beautiful truth.

On Tuesday, as we buried my ninety-seven-year-old grandmother, my friend Sari died of cancer. She was forty-seven years old, a wife and mother of two. It is a stretch to say Sari was my friend. I met her once last summer when I walked out of radiation and she was awaiting treatment, this beautiful young woman sitting in the lobby talking to David, who recognized and remembered her from his middle school years. But we traded our stories and exchanged a few emails: I'd had breast cancer twice, hers began elsewhere. By the time we met, it was in her bones.

My Grandpa David, for whom my son Ethan is named, died

when I was seventeen and a junior in high school, exactly the same age my daughter Ryan is now. I remember my grandfather fondly. His story of being an orphan along with his seven siblings, of hitching a ride while in uniform. I remember the tire shop that he owned and his bulldog named Daisy who lounged while he worked. I remember how he loved to bowl, played in a league and traveled for tournaments. I know that when he got married, my grandmother was eighteen and he was twenty-five, and I always remember him on his birthday. When I saw his gravestone at my grandmother's funeral revealing the date of his birth, I realized I've been one day off, but I remember him just the same. I remember the last time I heard his voice, which was the first time I'd heard it since the year that he died, when I dreamed of him while pregnant with my son, the son who I named in memory of him. My son, who has his eyes.

It is from my grandfather that my mother inherited the cancer gene, and my mother who passed it to me. The father of my mother who had breast cancer at fifty-four, then his granddaughter at thirty-five. And again last year at forty-three. The grandfather for whom my son is named, my son who has his eyes. The husband of my grandmother who died at ninety-seven but lived in perfect health. Fifty years longer than my beautiful friend.

I believe in the truth that my grandmother lived a long,

healthy life because she was such a positive person. I also believe it was luck.

I, too, divorce myself from negativity, eliminate stress wherever I can. I take care of myself and live my life right, with peace and light and love. And I know my friend Sari did, too.

We should all be so lucky to live our lives as long and as well and as healthy as my grandmother. We should all go out as peacefully. But all of us can't and all of us won't. We have to accept the hand we are dealt, to be grateful for all that we have. We have to believe and hope we'll be well, and not blame ourselves for if we are not.

My grandmother was a beautiful woman. My grandfather was a beautiful man. I have had cancer because of my mother, who had it because of him. Sari's life was taken by cancer, tragically short, our friendship shorter. Lengthy and brief, healthy and ill, I celebrate all of their lives.

Love Stacy

Please God let me go quickly
But not before my time
All around me I've seen death
And worse, I have seen dying

Six months of treatment, futile no less
A little girl sent home to die
A grandfather gone by a heart attack
Twenty years too shy

Affected by all of this
loss that surrounds me
My battle's been barely a cry
Losing my breasts now seems like nothing
So grateful to be here, not saying goodbye

JUNE 28, 2006

"Life is 10% of what happens to me and 90% of how I react to it."

—JOHN C. MAXWELL

August 17, 2015

Dear Cancer,

It's been one year. One year and two days since my last day of treatment. Since the day my doctor said I could start counting as a survivor. The days, the weeks, the months. A year.

One year. I am a one-year survivor. I am also a ten-year survivor. This month, August 2005, was when this all began. And then last year it began again. I am a one-year survivor and a ten-year survivor, but does the new outweigh the old? Does this second first year null the first nine, and void my original past?

I'm not sure I will ever assign a specific date to my

survivorship. I struggled with it altogether the first time around. But now there is no doubt. I AM A SURVIVOR.

There are so many dates I associate: the date of my mammogram gone awry; the weekend of waiting and then the news. The date of my bilateral mastectomy, forever etched on my body and mind. The day I received my diagnosis the second, shocking, earth shattering time. The scans and surgeries and chemo and hair loss. And then the end of radiation. I survived all of these things. One and ten years ago.

And that was the easy part.

Because then there's the anger. And also the fear. The dread of the future for knowing the past.

The guilt for the shame for the anger for the fear.

This summer I was feeling down, not in the deep but for a good long time, worry and sadness holding on. People I knew, both well and not, five young souls in the prime of their lives, all of them died this summer from cancer. Every one of them still in their forties, taken by this disease.

And here I am, alive to tell.

A new friend of mine saw an old picture of me and told me today about her surprise. She hadn't known I'd had long hair. She never knew me then.

I miss her, that girl. The old me. The then. That pretty young mom with the straight, long hair. I miss her. I miss me. I miss the then.

I miss her hair. I miss her health. I miss her freedom and joy.

I miss the way she loved to cook. I miss the way she loved to love. I miss the way she didn't worry. Does the new outweigh the old?

A few weeks ago I snapped out of my funk, but the tightrope is always there. I walk the balance between fear and hope, the past and the future, the old me and the new. These are the platforms of my life.

A ten percent chance of cancer recurrence, and ninety percent prospect of courage.

This past weekend, on the day of my one-year survivorship, I sat again inside a machine. But not a machine for radiation, a linear accelerator it's uncannily called. Instead it was one of a different kind, on an airplane flying home. On the day of my one-year survivorship, I was traveling with my family, on the trip we'd had to give up last year in exchange for re-starting my life. Perhaps by coincidence though I like to think not, we were able to grab a roundtrip to London—returning home on that same final day—and make up for last year's lost time.

I have grieved for the taken, been sad for the given, but here I am, alive to tell. With the gift of a year to feel all that confounds me, with hair and with health and with joy.

With hope for my future from knowing my past and because of the freedom to live.

Love Stacy

"The place of true healing is a fierce place. It's a giant place. It's a place of monstrous beauty and endless dark and glimmering light."

—CHERYL STRAYED

December 16, 2015

Dear Cancer,

It's been a year since my last scan, since the end of it all, and I am doing well.

I have not forgotten you. I think about you all the time. And also not so much.

Just wanted to check in and say *hi*.

Remind you that I'm still here.

Love Stacy

Love is why we are here.

January 13, 2016

Dear Cancer,

Today my yoga teacher talked about how our bodies regenerate every seven years. Ninety-five percent of our cells turn over. Only our brain and spine remain the same. Our core, who we are. Everything else has the chance to become anew.

I don't know, medically speaking, if this is correct. Or how, scientifically, anyone figured this out. But I don't care. I love the symbolism.

I love the symbolism of seven, like my birthday. Seven-seven-seventy. Clearly, seven is my lucky number.

Today is also my twenty-first anniversary. The denomination is not lost on me.

In fact, it is the very thing that makes today so special. More special than last year on my twentieth when I had just finalized all my treatment and testing but was not yet able to fully celebrate, still heavy with sadness and fear.

Today I am not. I am happy and light, and excited to celebrate my twenty-first anniversary. Our third renewal. Apropos for having been diagnosed with cancer, twice. Starting our life together, and then over, and then over again.

Even the years of my diagnosis, 2005 and 2014, each magically add up to seven, when the numerals are taken individually. I don't know if that is divine intervention or just the crazy math I do in my head. But it makes sense to me. And it makes me feel lucky.

Yes, instead of unlucky, I feel LUCKY. I was diagnosed, but I survived, twice. Both in the years whose count was seven.

Seven-seven-seventy.

Two + zero + zero + five. Two + zero + one + four.

Three times seven. Twenty-one.

All this time and I'm still here. From that day until now. From the day I was born through two diagnoses to twenty-one years of marriage.

I am still here.

And happy. And lucky. And loved.

Love Stacy

"Go confidently in the direction of your dreams. Live the life you have imagined."

March 4, 2016

Dear Cancer,

I was not going to mark this day. This day was supposed to be any old day. Even though two years ago on this day, I was diagnosed with cancer for the second time.

I am done with the anniversaries. Not because they pass without notice, and not because they aren't important. Every year, every day, every minute is worthy.

But I'm done with paying attention. I am done giving cancer a greeting card. No more hellos. No time for goodbyes. All I have time for is life.

But two years ago on this very day, four days before her sixteenth birthday, I was sitting next to my baby girl and

264 · STACY MIDDLEMAN

our life turned upside down. Right there in my daughter's room, my future hung heavy between us. In front of her eyes she saw the truth: the hard cold fact of uncertainty.

But today, everything is different. And today, everything is the same.

Today we got enormous news, but instead of bad it was good. Today we know our lives will change, but instead of bad, it is good.

Two years since that terrible day, and four days before her eighteenth birthday, TODAY, on this very same day, my daughter got into college. Not any old college, and not her first acceptance to college, but admittance to the only college she really wants to attend, the school she has dreamed of for years.

It's not just that her acceptance is wonderful news—it's the kind of thing that brought us to tears. It's the odd coincidence that instead of finding out in December, when we all thought that she would, or months ago when her friends found out, or week by week while we waited impatiently for the much-anticipated news, that she should find out on this very day, the day that once was marked.

The day that marked the change in our future has now

marked our future again. My beautiful girl is going to college, the college of her resolve. My baby bird is flying the nest and we're off for a new adventure, too. I am done with cancer. My life feels firm.

Today is the bookend to all our uncertainty. Our past is marked but our future is bright.

This day deserves a greeting card.

Love Stacy

Epilogue

"I have so much of you in my heart."
—JOHN KEATS

March 17, 2017

Dear Cancer,

Seven years in the making and suddenly it feels abrupt. We are officially moving to Austin. Knowing we've had one foot out the door feels somehow more sad than our final step. *Live for the moment, settle in.* Dear Cancer, lesson learned. Though perhaps if I hadn't looked so far ahead I would not have seen this day.

One great truth from emptying a house that took fifteen years to fill is that the only thing we really take is all the love that filled it. Memories are packed automatically. Everything else is just stuff.

We have had a wonderful life here. You will be missed. Our friends, this town, our house. You will always, always be in our heart. You will always be our home.

Love Stacy

* * *

A week or two before school let out one summer, when homework had subsided and softball and little league were over for the season, my family and I sat down to play a game of Monopoly. Not just good old ordinary Monopoly, but the new-fangled, up-to-date, everyone-has-millions *Monopoly Here and Now.* Apparently "America Has Voted!"—including my kids, who had asked for and received this version as one of their Hanukkah gifts—and the new game represents "A Modern Makeover for Today's Would-Be Billionaires" where the choice of game pieces includes a Starbucks coffee mug, a cell phone, a pack of McDonalds French fries, super-sized of course; an airplane, a dog, a New Balance tennis shoe, a lap-top computer and a Prius. My son Ethan, eleven at the time, was buying strategically and holding out for the goods. At four million dollars, Times Squares is the last and choicest of properties, where, coincidentally we had just recently visited, our family trip to New York serving as both a celebration of and gift to our daughter Ryan for her tenth birthday.

I was the first one to land on Community Chest, and my card read: "You appear on a TV morning news show to promote your new book. RECEIVE $1,000,000 IN ADDITIONAL ROYALTY FROM INCREASED SALES." We all shared a look. I asked them to wait a moment while I got up, left the room, and placed the card on my desk, never to be returned again to that brand-new box of Monopoly.

In the months preceding our trip, I had pursued an interest nagging at me for some time: to publish a collection of emails I had sent the previous year to family, friends, and ultimately an entire community during my first battle with breast cancer, and while in New York I had met with an agent who was interested in my story. My children had the opportunity to meet her—a real live person working in a building smack in the middle of crazy Times Square—and they understood and were excited about my new project.

Time passed, life got in the way, and my desire to publish those emails waned. And then in 2014 I was re-diagnosed and compelled again to write. For years I have longed to publish my writings—both my emails from 2005 and these Facebook posts—not only to express my experience with cancer but how sharing it, in part, is what really saved me.

That Community Chest card, which still resides on a bulletin board just above my desk, told me something. There was more to my future. And I had a story to tell. It wasn't so much a wish fulfilled as it was the luck of the draw, but my life has been filled with that sort of coincidence and good fortune, and it was yet another reminder of the odd and enlightening timing of things.

✳ ✳ ✳

My intention with this memoir was to tell a complete story, from beginning to end, about who I am and how all of this came to be. Why I knew to get checked and how, with my first diagnosis, I instinctively coped. And then, after having been through it once, how I somehow missed the signs, and ended up doing this twice.

But life—a whole life—is complicated, and so I decided that all that matters is all right here, exactly as I went through it, the second time around. The poems scattered throughout this book are a nod to my emails from a decade ago. What happened all those years ago—my diagnosis and bilateral mastectomy, and the things I wrote to help me cope—and what has happened since then—my ignorance about breast cancer and the arrogance that I could outsmart it—all add up to *Dear Cancer, Love Stacy*. The girl with the rage with the words on the page. With the hope and the luck to survive.

It is difficult to present in book form the interaction that occurred by sharing these passages online. *Dear Cancer, Love Stacy* was an outlet for me, but as a Facebook page I also knew it would be a receptacle, a place for people to reach out and support me.

Though my posts generated many comments, I made a conscious decision from the beginning not to engage publicly—no comments or likes on my behalf. I did not want to acknowledge, inadvertently or otherwise, one friend or follower over another. This was something I needed to do—to write and to share—without wanting to create something else to manage while struggling through my treatment.

A large part of its power, however, was the way people did in fact respond, with views and likes and commentary. The attention I received, an outpouring of support not only for my journey but also for the way in which it was shared, contributed in many ways to my healing. As much as these posts were written for myself, for my own release and sanity, the fact that people cared, and were moved, and could relate to my experience or begin to understand things which they never could before—that I may have helped anyone in any way—this in turn helped me. The distraction became a necessity. The necessity created a space for healing.

And on the subject of healing ...

Writing was easy when the pain was acute, but as treatment concluded, my writing slowed. Healing, however, is a process. It is not linear or neat or terminable. It is winding, and messy, and most of all, it is never complete. It has been more than a decade since my first diagnosis and bilateral mastectomy. I thought I had recovered, until my second diagnosis taught me the truth about cancer: that survivorship is forever. For as long as you are lucky enough to be alive. My healing is ongoing, still.

I have come to accept many things on this journey, not just the things I already knew: that life is beautiful and painful and wonderful and unfair, and that anyone at any time can be taken from us. What I really came to understand was that *that anyone* could have been *me*. Accepting my death became a part of my life: what it would mean for me, and for my husband and our beautiful kids, and what it would mean for the rest of their lives. I have learned to accept that even without me, they would survive. It would not be fair, but they would be okay.

I do not know what the future holds, both in terms of my health and theirs. My children will need to be tested, to find out if they are BRCA positive. It is a burden I carry every day, wondering and waiting until the time is right. Knowing I will have to acknowledge their fear and uncertainty, or worse, bear witness to their suffering and pain. Reminding myself that no matter what, even if they carry the mutation which I could not help but pass on, we all will be okay. And believing, believing, believing, that in the sharp light of unfairness, there is hope.

In 2005, when I was first diagnosed with breast cancer, BRCA testing had only been around for ten years. The

BRCA-1 and BRCA-2 mutations, discovered in 1994 and 1995 respectively, were relatively new to science and genetics testing was, for all intents and purposes, still a novelty. BRCA testing was one of the first genetic tests to become available for clinical use in October of 1995, but awareness of the test and the willingness to undergo it was inhibited by patients' concerns about confidentiality, inability to pay, and perceived access to genetics counseling[12]—to say nothing of what to do with the information once it was received. I, for one, did not know enough to seek out testing until after I was diagnosed. Insurance did not cover the $3,000 testing fee, but we wanted as many answers as we could get before finalizing my decision for treatment, which was to remove both breasts when only one had developed cancer. It was the right thing to do, both the testing and the bilateral mastectomy, but even with the information I was given, it turned out not to be enough. I did not know what I was up against, until I was up against it again.

Incidentally, the first thing I did upon my second diagnosis, before I started treatment or began writing on my Facebook page, was to google BRCA. I needed to understand what I had missed, why I had missed it, and what I could do to prevent such crises in the future. I did not understand that being a carrier meant that I would always be at risk.

---

12   Cho, M.K. et al. "Commercialization of *BRCA1/2* Testing: Practitioner Awareness and Use of a New Genetic Test." *American journal of medical genetics* 83.3 (1999): 157–163. Print.

That even in spite of having a bilateral mastectomy, I still remained at risk for a secondary breast cancer. I believed so strongly that this could never happen again that I ignored what should have been obvious signs.

In 2012, two years before my second diagnosis, and seven years after my first, an organization was founded to provide people like me—families with a history of BRCA—with the information and research we so desperately need. The Basser Center for BRCA, part of Penn Medicine's Abramson Cancer Center, is the only center in the world solely devoted to BRCA-related cancers. By creating a centralized place for finding breakthroughs and discoveries, Basser Center has revolutionized research and patient education for individuals living with BRCA-1 and BRCA-2 mutations. Not only did I come to understand how important it is to know your BRCA status, I had also found my cause. Basser's efforts may hold the key to the future of so many of us affected, my children and their children included.

Additionally, a few months into treatment, a filmmaker found my page and asked if she could turn my story about cancer and the way I wrote about it into a documentary. *What did I have to lose?* I asked myself. Part of facing my fear was pursuing fearlessness, which is what it took to be put on film. It made perfect sense to connect my story with its cause, and gave me the opportunity to channel my pain into something good, something bigger than myself. We were able to connect the project with something that may help prevent others from suffering in the future, by raising awareness and support for Basser Center. Through a serendipitous series of events, I found myself right where I needed to be, rising to the call.

In the years since my diagnosis, there were other fortuitous moments as well. I did, in fact, meet Cheryl Strayed, whose story about losing her mother to cancer and finding her way back to this world resonated strongly with me. That I had written about her writing and had mentioned that I hoped to meet her one day was ever more the mystery. A writing conference she was leading, "The Story You Have to Tell," curiously came to my attention while I was in treatment, and in another leap of faith, I signed up. It was on this trip, purposely out of my comfort zone, where I had an epiphany about my life.

On the final day of the conference, the moderator of the week-long event asked us to leave the room and walk silently outside, toward a meditation circle. There I stood, shielded under cerulean sky, so blue it seemed crisp. But it was humid and warm, and the humidity had my hair in waves, unfamiliar curls I was still learning to accept. Or ignore, depending on my mood.

I was alone in Maui, in the middle of an exquisitely mani-
cured wide open space, soft and beautiful and green. It was
in this beautiful place where I stepped into the labyrinth, a
walking circle situated in the center of the field, behind a
garden with its giant statue of Buddha. Just like the curated
landscape it flanked, the walking path was meticulously
kept, its borders made of black crushed granite, the path-
way filled with light gray stones. This walking path was a
work of art.

I had never walked through a meditation circle, nor seen
one before this week. In all my years of practicing yoga, I
had never heard of such a thing. A walking labyrinth is a
patterned path made up of concentric circles, arranged in
such a way that you are led through a series of curves until
you reach the center, at which point you are led back out
again. Unlike a maze which may have dead ends, a labyrinth
leads in only one direction, offering one way in and one
way out, leaving no problems to be solved. I noticed the
circle throughout my stay, but did not think to take the
time to walk its graceful path.

Slowly and with a calculated pace, I entered. Now that I
was leaving this place, I wanted to savor the experience.
Strolling leisurely among the stones, I felt soothed by my
steps, attentive to the rocks below, each one articulated
under my feet. Even in my thoughtful state, I noticed each

turn as it came about, how the path meandered around the perimeter, toward the center and eventually out, but not in a direct manner. The labyrinth had led me back and forth in ways I could not predict.

As I passed through the circle, in, around and out, something inside me began to shift. A clarity came over me, something so intense it felt like a revelation. By the time I walked out I was overcome and weeping beyond control. In the metaphor of the circle, by the act of walking its winding path, I saw a vision of my life.

This is my life. This walk, this labyrinth ... this is it. *This is life.* Every moment, every turn, every step we notice and each one overlooked ... every instance of my life was reflected in those rocks.

By the simple act of walking our movement propels us forward, yet the path leads the way. Sometimes it is easy. Once in a while we trip and fall. Sometimes we know where we are going. Other times we are moved along in unexpected ways.

Life is a journey, and in this circle I had symbolically taken the trek. We enter, we walk, we exit. We are born, we live, we die. This was the passage through life, the path that every single one of us takes, no matter the substance of our experience or the length of our time on this earth.

Suddenly, and wrenched with tears, I was overwhelmed with peace, an acceptance of my life given as a whole. The labyrinth was my life complete: beginning, middle, and end. I saw my past. I sensed my future. I envisioned every step I had taken, and all the steps I had yet to take, though I didn't know how many were left. And somehow that was okay.

Hawaii was not a spiritual quest. I had not left my family and traveled alone in search of the meaning of life. I did not think I needed to heal. Instead I had come for a writing workshop, hoping to improve my skills. For the better part of that previous year I had spent my time with my words, not for the sake of telling my story, but in order to survive.

On that last day of my solo trip, everything became illuminated. The labyrinth was my guiding light. Here I was, on my sacred journey. In the midst of my given life. Walking on the very path of the story I had to tell.

So this is where my story ends. Somewhere in the middle. I have been changed profoundly, by cancer and by love. My writing has ceased, naturally. My healing continues, as it must. No day is taken for granted, and there is important work ahead. To find a cure for this awful disease. To put an end to the BRCA mutation. To be there for my children, to live my life to its fullest and continue to fight the good fight. Like a girl. And a motherfucker.

Author's Note

At the moment of my second diagnosis, we were deep in the throes of designing a house. Our dream for a change of scenery when the kids were finished with high school was immediately put on hold. David was adamant about planning our future while I was afraid to embrace it. But all things are temporary, including our halt, so we forged on through, in the midst—and in spite—of my treatment. I do not take for granted any of it: that we have been lucky enough to fulfill our dreams, the greatest one of being alive.

It should be mentioned that while I was gathering ideas on Pinterest for my new home, I became as equally enthralled with quotes as I was for inspirational pictures of flooring and bathrooms. It was from this collection—my online bulletin board of uplifting thoughts—that I added an epigraph to each of my posts, one that seemed to match my current sentiment and not the other way around.

In some cases, the quotes were attributed to an actual person, while others seemed to have been created for websites, e-cards, memes and the like, and shared in the public domain. The World Wide Web is a tricky place but a place that gave me hope, and so I used it to my advantage. When I decided to publish this work beyond the scope of Facebook, I honestly did not know where to begin to fairly credit the authors of these words. All such quotes have been researched and acknowledged to the best of my ability, and uncredited sayings and expressions were used with honest intentions. I apologize for any misuse or mistakes.

Acknowledgments

There are so many people and places in my life for whom I am so very grateful, from my first diagnosis until now. If any should go unmentioned, it is not for lack of gratitude and love.

Thank you to every single person who read and regarded my emails and Facebook page, for your positive energy, love and support.

Facebook, for giving me a place for my rage, and Pinterest to make it seem clever.

My extensive team of doctors, nurses and staff, for your compassion and care, and for devoting your lives to saving others', Dr. Jenny Chang and Dr. Jeffrey Friedman in particular.

Houston Methodist Hospital, for my past.

Basser Center for BRCA, for the future.*

My parents Robin Beerman, Rhoda and Stan Linnick, and Shelly and Ed Middleman for giving me and guiding me through life.

Joanne Brownstein Jarvi, my agent, for believing in me since the very beginning. You are a survivor, too.

Stacey Summers, for finding, filming and producing *Dear Cancer, Love Stacy* and helping me connect the dots in so many important ways. **

YogaOne Studios for being my sanctuary, with special mention to Albina and Roger Rippy, Jannell Brown, Liz Ching and Lee Moffett. In every class and with every teacher, your studio helped me heal.

Every one of my children's friends, their families, The Emery/Weiner School and Beth Yeshurun Day School for looking out for my kids when they, too, were getting through.

My friends, however near or far, in distance and in life:

Marris Goldberg, Susie Raizner and many, many others for being there the first time.

Adina Chirogianis, Alyssa Rosenthal, and everyone else for being there the second.

Debbie Natelson, Laurie Cohen and Leora Hamberger Elliot, for being there forever.

Trayci Kessel Handelman, for giving me perspective when I needed it most.

John Scott Black, for lending your voice to my cause.

Jennifer Black, for your friendship and advice, all of it constructive.

Jennifer Oakley, for your encouragement and belief.

Teresa and Lenny Friedman, for being my biggest fans.

David Pulaski, for saying you'd take the bullet for me and meaning it;

Jayme (and Scott) Morgan for understanding my wicked sense of humor;

Rebeca (and Greg) Huddle for your friendship and brilliance; and

Elisabeth (and Stuart) Wallock for your open-hearted light. Thank you all for sitting with me through chemo when there are better ways to spend a day.

Elia Graves Pulaski for being the best damn hair stylist a girl could ask for. I am lucky to call you my friend.

Everyone whom we have loved in Houston; there are far too many names to name.

Our dear friends in Austin who made us want to make the move, especially these few:

Cindy and Adrian Lufschanowski, pharmacist extraordinaire and dachshund lovers to boot;

Emmy and Stephen Sunshine, for making me laugh and having my back; and

Amy and Adam Mosier, for becoming family and fighting the fight.

Ethan and Ryan, my beautiful children.
Thank you for being my everything.
And David, my husband.
For everything.

Proceeds from Dear Cancer, Love Stacy
will benefit breast cancer research.

*For more information about the BRCA mutation
and Basser Center for BRCA, visit
www.basser.org

**For information about the documentary
Dear Cancer, Love Stacy
produced by Poppy Pro Productions, visit
www.dearcancerlovestacy.com

Visit Stacy Middleman's Facebook page:
www.Facebook.com/Dear-Cancer-Love-Stacy

About the Author

Stacy Middleman is a proud mom, truth-talker and two-time survivor of breast cancer. She loves good people, bad words, art, yoga and dachshunds. Stacy was born and raised in Houston, Texas, where she lived with her family for twenty-two years. She recently moved to Austin with her husband, David, and their dog, Ace.

93971441R00174

Made in the USA
Columbia, SC
24 April 2018